KU-031-364

strategies for those inevitable bleak moments, and for anyone who wants to understand what cancer sufferers are going through'

– Julia Palca, Chairman, Macmillan Cancer Support
and cancer survivor

'People living with cancer need clear, down-to-earth and empowering advice to move beyond their diagnosis. This book is an important tool in that process'

– Laura Lee, Chief Executive, Maggie's Cancer Caring Centres

'This book sensitively addresses the ongoing issues that so many people face when moving forward after treatment for breast cancer. Importantly, it enables readers to see that they are not alone in their experience'

– Dr Emma Pennery, Clinical Director, Breast Cancer Care

'A wonderful book. Recovery from cancer does not stop when the chemotherapists and surgeons have said good luck and goodbye. This is not only full of excellent advice but advice given in the clearest and most practical way'

– Sir Peter Stothard, Editor of *The Times Literary Supplement* and
Patron of the Neuroendocrine Tumour Patient Foundation

'This is an enormously readable and practical guide which will be invaluable in helping people coming through the storm of cancer to understand their feelings and regain a sense of mental well-being. It dispels the myth that getting over cancer "should" be a cause for celebration, and instead provides reassurance and realistic strategies for coming to terms with the many challenges that recovery from cancer can bring'

– Geraldine Mynors, Development Director of the Patient
Information Forum

life. This book should help them to recognise their fears and hopes. It is really a companion that they must have'

– Dr Bashir Qureshi, Emeritus Vice President of the
Royal Society of Public Health, Vice President,
GP & PHC Section of the Royal Society of Medicine,
2012 BMA Medical Book Awards Programme

'This excellent guide offers simple, practical ways to tackle worries, exhaustion, anger and depression . . . as well as simple but effective self-help exercises and tips throughout'

– *Nursing Standard*

'a useful library resource for primary care nurses, and patients and families would benefit from owning a copy for its supportive approach'

– *Primary Health Care*

The
Cancer Survivor's
Companion

*Practical ways to cope with
your feelings after cancer*

Dr Frances Goodhart and Lucy Atkins

piatkus

To friendship, without which this book –
and so much more – would not exist.

PIATKUS

First published in Great Britain in 2011 by Piatkus
This paperback edition published in 2013 by Piatkus
Reprinted 2013, 2014

A CIP catalogue record for this book is available from the British Library.

The case studies featured in the book are based on cases from Dr Frances Goodhart's
clinical work. All names and some details have been changed to protect the
anonymity of the people Dr Goodhart worked with.

The recommendations given in this book are solely intended as education and information. Check with your doctor before changing or stopping
any treatments or medications, and keep your doctor informed of all
treatments that you are receiving.

ISBN 978-0-7499-5490-1

Designed and Typeset in Aldus and The Sans by Paul Saunders
Printed and bound in Great Britain by
Clays Ltd, St Ives plc

Papers used by Piatkus are from well-managed forests
and other responsible sources.

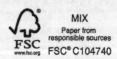

Piatkus
An imprint of
Little, Brown Book Group
100 Victoria Embankment
London EC4Y 0DY

An Hachette UK Company
www.hachette.co.uk

www.piatkus.co.uk

CONTENTS

ACKNOWLEDGEMENTS

First, enormous thanks to all the cancer survivors who were brave and determined enough to seek emotional help. Your stories, struggles, triumphs and experiences are the heart of this book. Many thanks go to Bernie Byrne and Katie Tait from Maggie's Centres for their help, ideas and enthusiasm. Thanks to Macmillan clinical psychologists Dr Heather Wells and Dr Nicola Taylor for reading, commenting and encouraging the early drafts; to Dr Simon Dupont, Consultant Clinical Psychologist for his support; to Dr Emma Pennery of Breast Cancer Care and Tracy Williams of Macmillan Cancer Support for invaluable expertise; to Trisha Goddard for taking time out to talk to and inspire us and to Cal Smith for great comments.

Frances: and thanks to Jim, Josie, Beatrice and Kitty, with love and apologies for hogging the computer.

Lucy: thanks to John, Izzie, Sam and Ted for the many times I've ignored you while writing this.

INTRODUCTION

> ❛I thought that getting my diagnosis and making it
> through treatment would be the toughest bits of cancer.
> I had no idea that coping with life afterwards would be so
> tough – and scary. Sometimes, life after the all-clear feels
> as hard as anything that came before.❜
>
> **CARL, 53, KIDNEY CANCER SURVIVOR**

The storm of cancer

Before cancer, you're sailing along in generally fair weather.
You're travelling in one direction. You have maps, navigation
aids and provisions. You might even be part of a flotilla – you
and some other boats, sailing in the same direction at the same
speed. Life is fine, good even.

Then a massive storm hits – cancer.

Your boat is seriously damaged. Maybe parts of it are lost
or broken. Your maps and provisions are swept overboard. In
the eye of the storm, you lose all sense of direction. Your main
terror is that the boat will sink.

Then your cancer care team appear. They are your lifeboat;
your rescuers. They attach ropes, patch your boat up and
keep it afloat; they come alongside you, and take control of

the steering and direction. Slowly, they tow you back to port. Sometimes this journey towards the port is even stormier than the catastrophe itself. But you know you are not alone – you have the lifeboat staff, you make a good team.

As the lifeboat tows your boat back to port you see friends and family on the shore waving and cheering. They are so relieved to have you back.

But then your boat just stops.

You are not quite back in port. You can see the lights, and your happy loved ones. But you're moored just outside the mouth of the harbour. Then your lifeboat, and its team, goes. They drop the ropes into the water and sail away.

You might think: I can get back to port on my own. You've been there before, after all. And you can see it, right there, quite close. But it all feels different now. Your boat is still damaged. You need time for repairs. You need to get a new map and provisions. And you keep looking at the sky – is the storm coming back? You listen constantly, obsessively, to the weather forecast – you hear reports of hurricanes. They may be far away, but you can't stop yourself from feeling that they are coming for you.

This boat analogy may seem long-winded, but it accurately describes what surviving cancer can feel like – does feel like – for many people. You may feel stranded, but this book is here to help. It's your map, your repair kit, and your navigator.

Who are we?

Dr Frances Goodhart: I am an NHS consultant clinical psychologist with twenty years' experience of working with individuals and families who are coping with life-threatening illnesses. While working as a Macmillan consultant clinical psychologist, many of the cancer survivors I saw (as well as their loved ones, and sometimes even their healthcare teams) would ask me to recommend a good book. I was always stumped. There was no single book that would explain why reaching the successful end of cancer treatment can throw up such complicated, difficult emotions. And there was no professional, practical and problem-solving guide that I could recommend. Talking one day to Lucy Atkins, a well-known health writer, and close friend of mine for twenty-five years, the answer became clear to both of us: if there wasn't a good book for cancer survivors then we'd have to write one. Here it is. The case studies featured are based on cases I have come across in my work. All names and some details have been changed to protect the anonymity of the people I worked with.

Lucy Atkins: I have been an author and health writer for fifteen years. As a writer for newspapers such as the *Guardian* or *Sunday Times*, I often have to translate complicated information from doctors, scientists and other specialists into readable and usable messages. This book is rooted in evidence-based research and years of clinical expertise. But who wants dry complexity – least of all, post-cancer? My job has been to make this book friendly, sensible, practical – and most of all human. The kind of companion you don't mind spending time with.

Life after cancer

The idea that the successful end of treatment for cancer brings relief, peace and celebrations just isn't true for many cancer survivors. It can be quite tricky even to work out quite **when** you have finished your treatment. Everyone will have a different moment when they feel that they're no longer on the treadmill and it's time to start 'getting back to normal'. The problem is that when this moment comes it can actually make you feel more lost, alone and worried than ever before. It can be the time when all those tricky feelings, that have been mounting up as you go through the trauma of diagnosis and treatment, really kick in.

Right now, you may be facing major physical and practical challenges. Or you may just be feeling slightly lost and worried. But one thing's for sure: for every person who sails back into port after cancer and carries on as before, there's another person (or several) left adrift: confused, worried and tired.

Myths and expectations

'Finishing my breast cancer treatment reminded me of when I became a mother,' says Marilyn, 62, a breast cancer survivor. 'I felt as if this was what I had been working towards for months. But when I got there it was harder than I expected, and I thought that everyone else was doing a better job than me. It took me ages to realise that doing my best was good enough.'

Cancer survival is a bit like becoming a parent. It's loaded with myths and expectations. Just as new parents often believe that they'll feel instant, automatic love for their newborn, people at the end of cancer treatment often expect to feel overjoyed, excited, fit and ready to lead a 'more meaningful life'.

Of course, some new parents do fall instantly in love with their newborn, and then sail through the nappies and sleepless nights on a cloud of bliss. And some people – you may know one – do come through cancer, its treatment and the aftermath, with barely a wobble.

But most don't.

The end of treatment is a new life phase – a huge change. You're bound to have ups and downs – sometimes major ones. You may not really want to admit this to anyone. And you may wish you didn't feel this way. It might take longer than you think to adjust. But one thing is clear: you're definitely not alone.

As Roger, 68, prostate cancer survivor, puts it, 'You feel weakened physically and psychologically and rebuilding your strength doesn't happen overnight. You may be strong, but you're not superhuman, are you?'

Cancer brings an enormous shift in anyone's life. And it can feel so sudden. Looking back, many cancer survivors, even if the diagnosis was long and drawn-out, say they were struck by the speed between diagnosis and treatment. 'It was a whirlwind,' says Carol, 51, lung cancer survivor. 'I was given my diagnosis on Friday, told to consider my treatment options over the weekend, went back to the consultant on Monday, and was having surgery by Wednesday.'

When all this is happening, everything feels urgent. You're making medical decisions; trawling the internet; navigating the hospital system; explaining things to family, friends and colleagues; packing bags; making complicated arrangements – often in a matter of days.

Then there are weeks or months of treatment: surgery, chemotherapy, radiotherapy, hormonal management – and their myriad side effects. 'I was on automatic,' Carol remembers. 'It was as if I shut down emotionally. I didn't cry, I didn't wail, I just used my professional skills – I am an accountant and I love structure – to plan out the next stage of my life.'

While this is going on, many people do find a strength and resilience they didn't know they had. Cancer is the 'enemy' and they're going to tackle it with everything they've got. Some people develop a 'fighting spirit' – they find out all the details of the treatment plan, work in close partnership with the medical team, set themselves small, realistic daily targets, enlist and accept support, understand their treatment, ask questions, face the answers full on. People praise their 'courage' and 'strength'.

Other people put themselves in the hands of the medical team. They don't want much information. They follow the team's advice. They don't feel the same level of responsibility, with all the pressures that come with it. People praise them for the quiet, peaceful and accepting way they are coping with the trauma.

However you coped; when treatment ends you face a set of different challenges. If you're the 'fighting spirit' type, your 'enemy' might suddenly seem less clear. It can be hard to find information. You are physically run down after all that fighting. This is when the emotional after-effects of cancer really kick in.

If you're the quieter type, you may find it really hard that your team has suddenly gone. You're on your own. You might feel isolated, maybe abandoned and vulnerable. Again, all this hits you just when you're physically and emotionally exhausted. It's incredibly tough.

No one is suggesting here that you shouldn't be allowed to celebrate the end of treatment. You, together with your medical team, have achieved something fantastic. Many survivors do get moments of elation. But it tends to be more complicated than cracking open the champagne and settling back into your old life.

What this book won't do

You may be struggling with lots of medical and practical issues, along with all these unexpected emotions. There might be long-term physical effects from the cancer or its treatment. Maybe you are still making decisions about things like reconstructive surgery or fertility treatment. You might also be struggling with your finances, your rights at work, your insurance policies or other upsetting and time-consuming practicalities. These are important post-cancer issues, huge in your life right now, but they are not what this book is about. Other books tackle these practical issues. The aim here is to concentrate on your feelings.

We also won't be giving any lectures in positive thinking. We aren't going to ask you to think of cancer as a gift. We aren't going to suggest that you see yourself as lucky or blessed. We are going to ask you to explore your thoughts and question whether what you are saying to yourself is true, realistic and fair. We'll encourage you to do this even when you want to curl up under the duvet and shut the whole world out. But we won't – ever – tell you to look on the bright side.

'If one more person tells me how lucky I am to be through my cancer when I've lost my breast, my hair, my confidence and my sense of who I am, I think I'm going to explode!' says Dawn, 44, breast cancer survivor.

What this book will do for you

This book will help you with the **emotions** of cancer survival. We will give you simple, practical ways to tackle things like worries, fatigue, anger or depression. These are the feelings that can hold you back and stop you from adjusting to life after cancer.

Coping with emotions doesn't mean getting rid of them. You're not going to read this book and magically enter a 'feelings-free zone' – far from it. But you will learn how to understand, explore and challenge your difficult post-cancer emotions.

None of this, incidentally, involves 'wallowing', 'navel gazing' or 'dredging things up'. We just give you concrete, easy to follow strategies (based on scientific research), along with tips and ideas to help you cope.

These strategies won't work overnight, and they won't stop you from feeling upset at times. Some of the exercises won't be right for you at this point, but they might be a bit later on, so it's always worth coming back to things – even if you thought they were unhelpful the first time around.

Who is this book for?

This book is a useful resource for any survivor – whether it's days, months or years since your treatment ended. It should be helpful whether you're feeling a little bit daunted, or completely adrift.

It will also be valuable for the families and friends of cancer survivors. If your loved one's treatment has ended, you're likely to be going through surprisingly similar emotions yourself. You might feel shell-shocked, confused, worried (and maybe even annoyed) by your loved one's reaction to what you hoped would be 'the end' of this cancer thing. You need support too – you've also been through so much – and this book is your valuable starting point. We'll give you ways to understand what you're both going through, and ideas for coping (and helping).

Finally, this book is also aimed at health professionals. It will help you to recognise, perhaps in more detail, or more systematically, what happens to your patients after they close the clinic door. It will also give you strategies to suggest to people if they need your advice, either immediately after treatment ends, or much later, when they come back for check-ups and you notice that they're struggling.

In short, this book is your companion, supporting and advising as you move your life onwards. Your boat may not feel the same and the landscape may have changed, but it's still yours. You can do this.

CHAPTER ONE

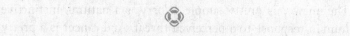

WORRIES

> 6 My husband and I always said we'd go away on holiday once the treatment was all over. But when my treatment finished it didn't feel like it was all over, not to me. I worried that I couldn't organise a holiday like I did before. But worst of all, I worried that it was almost asking for trouble to celebrate. 9

BERYL, 71, UTERINE CANCER SURVIVOR

What's so worrying?

It is extraordinarily common to feel worried after cancer. Worries can keep you awake at night, stop you eating, give you butterflies in your stomach, make you snappy, panicky, fretful or just a bit uneasy. They can range from out and out panic attacks to a persistent sense of vagueness or nervousness. This can go on for a very long time after cancer treatment ends – sometimes years (if you don't know what to do about it).

But why?

The answer is pretty simple. Worry is a natural, instinctive human response to a perceived threat. And cancer is a pretty huge threat, by anyone's standards.

Worries during diagnosis and treatment

When you are first diagnosed with cancer your whole world changes. You are instantly forced to start making decisions. You're bombarded by treatment options, percentages, research trials and outcome studies. You have to make choices, filter information and engage with complicated issues. This, obviously, can be really worrying and stressful. 'I'm a head teacher and spend my working life making difficult choices and decisions', says Malcolm, 57, oral cancer survivor. 'But when I had to decide about what treatment to have for my cancer, it was as if my mind had turned to jelly. I couldn't remember what the doctor had just told me five minutes before. All options seemed so frightening, and I simply felt incapable of making any rational decision. My wife and my clinical nurse specialist had to hold my hand and coax me through the whole process.'

Next, during your treatment phase, you have to cope with what can be dreadful symptoms and an alien environment: hospital wards, theatre recovery rooms, radiotherapy machines and chemotherapy suites. You're bombarded by frightening sights, sounds and sensations; by needles, nausea and noise. Again, all this can make you anxious. Sometimes it's the smallest things that set you off. 'The first time I saw the skull and crossbones on the door to the radiotherapy room,' says Paul, 65, colon cancer survivor, 'I wondered what on earth I was doing there and I very nearly ran.'

But all this is over now. It's in the past. You've got through cancer. Your treatment is done and you're putting your life back together. Why, then, are you still worrying?

When worries won't go away

Right now you are probably trying to pick up the pieces of your life. People might talk about your strength and bravery. You might have moments when you want to yell from the rooftops about how amazing you are to have got through this. But there are probably also times when the threat of cancer still feels very real. You don't feel the same certainty about life any more. Your future seems unknown and, perhaps at times, very scary indeed.

During treatment you actually got quite used to the hospital environment and your medical team. It can feel weird not to have them around any more, for reassurance and support. There's nothing to 'fight' now either: your treatment is finished. And after months, or maybe years of struggle, your coping skills are probably at a low ebb. Basically, you're exhausted.

Ending cancer treatment is a huge life event. It's as big as diagnosis and treatment. But nobody seems to recognise this. Your team sends you off, telling you to get on with your life. Your friends and family expect you to be delighted. You're supposed to put the whole thing behind you.

However, the focus of your life has changed completely – and change isn't often easy to handle.

When is worrying a problem?

Worry only really becomes a problem when it starts to interfere with your life. And you might be surprised just how many people this happens to after cancer.

> **PROBLEMATIC WORRIES**
>
> If you:
>
> - feel preoccupied by your worries, can't get them out of your head

- can't focus on other things because you're so busy worrying
- worry over small, everyday matters as well as big, important ones
- wish you could stop worrying so much

...then you'll really benefit from some of the help and ideas in this chapter.

It's OK to worry

Cancer survivors are often ashamed of their anxieties. They think that worrying might be a sign of weakness – maybe a bit 'pathetic' or 'silly'. They feel they owe it to the medical staff or their friends and family – everyone who's helped them to get through this – to be strong and happy. They also worry that they are making things worse by fretting: maybe holding up their own recovery. Often, they don't admit, even to their nearest and dearest, quite how worried they are. It's a lonely place to be.

Virtually every cancer survivor goes through this. For some people, the post-cancer anxiety is short lived. But the majority find their worries much harder to shake off. For many cancer survivors worry becomes really problematic – it stops them getting on with their life.

COMMON POST-CANCER WORRIES

- I'm scared that the cancer may come back. (The fear that 'something feels wrong'.)
- I can't get it out of my head. (Scary or traumatic memories

and thoughts about diagnosis and treatment keep popping back into my mind.)

- I'm worried about family and friends. (Am I putting too much strain on them? Do they understand what I'm going through? Why aren't we communicating better?)

- I'm worried about the future. (How will I cope if I always feel this way? What will I do with the rest of my life? Will I ever feel like 'me' again?)

- I'm not coping. (Life has changed; I'm struggling with side effects or other changes after treatment; I feel burdened, alone, sometimes overwhelmed.)

CASE STUDY

Bill, 49, testicular cancer survivor

Check-up anxiety

Bill is a married taxi driver and father of three. His treatment finished five years ago. 'For fifty weeks of the year I'm fine,' he told me in our first session, 'but for the two weeks before my annual check-up I feel like a nervous wreck all over again. I go inwards, stop talking to my wife, get irritable with the kids and just find myself wondering: What if it has come back?'

Going into the hospital waiting area was difficult for Bill: just the paint colour, the smell, the noises brought that terrible year back to him. It made him feel as if his cancer was yesterday, not five years ago. 'It makes me so cross with myself,' he said, 'I should be beyond this.'

→

First, I asked Bill what he'd say to a friend in a similar situation. Would he tell them that they 'should be beyond this' or would he say 'It's natural to worry, no one could go back into that setting and not experience some anxiety'?

Many of us are great at supporting other people, but those skills go out the window when it comes to our own worries ('I'm so weak/pathetic/silly'). We set ourselves harsh, unfair or unrealistic targets ('I should be doing X or Y by now...'). This just adds to the stress.

In fact, Bill was doing incredibly well. He'd found a way to make cancer part of his past for fifty weeks of the year. But he was also expecting a lot of himself.

With his next check-up approaching, Bill tried talking to himself as if he were talking to his own best friend. He reassured himself, and accepted his worries, instead of getting at himself for being 'weak'. This process, he said, made him feel much calmer – and more accepting of his own anxiety.

I also worked with Bill to understand the fear itself: What if it has come back? To unpick this fear, Bill asked himself these questions:

- *What evidence do I have that there is any problem?*

- *Do I have physical concerns, or it is just the clinic appointment letter that has made me anxious?*

- *Have I felt this way before, but the cancer had not come back?*

The answers Bill gave to these questions made him realise that his fears were not always completely balanced and realistic. Bill realised how his worries pushed his thoughts to extremes – making them frightening, and heightening his worry.

Understanding your worries

It isn't self-indulgent to take some time to think about your worries. It's essential.

If you can understand more about how worry works in general, and unpick what is really getting to you, then you stand a far better chance of coping. You can learn simple ways to reduce your worry, stress or panicky feelings. You aren't going to erase all worry from your life – sadly, none of us can do that. But you will be able to manage unwanted thoughts and emotions so that they don't get the better of you.

HOW WORRY WORKS

Worry, like all emotions, is made up of four key elements:

1. Your thoughts
2. Your feelings
3. Your behaviour
4. Your body

Basically, if you learn simple ways to manage each of these four elements, then you will start to feel far more in control – and far less worried.

Worried feelings

When you feel threatened by something, or overloaded with demands that you don't think you can cope with, then you might feel any or all of these emotions:

- stress
- worry
- fear
- panic

- anxiety
- edginess
- confusion.

These feelings might build up slowly, or they might suddenly burst out. They might feel a bit vague, or they might feel really intense. It doesn't really matter what you call these feelings – anxiety, stress, worry. They all basically mean the same thing (see page 36 for information about panic, which works in a slightly different way).

There are two things that really do matter:

1. You will not always feel this way.

2. There are things that you can do right now to start feeling better.

How to manage your worried feelings

Stop worrying! Don't feel anxious! Control your stress! It's easier said than done, isn't it? But you don't have to miraculously change the way you feel overnight. You just have to learn to understand your feelings better so you can cope with them more effectively.

The first step is simple. You learn to identify exactly when your emotional state changes – pinpoint the moment when you go from feeling basically OK, to feeling worried, uptight or stressed out.

'I'd been very calm, having a nice day putting some photos in an album, when I heard on the radio that Bobby Robson had died,' says Arthur, 71, bowel cancer survivor. 'I was so upset after that; I couldn't settle to anything, I was on edge for hours.'

Noticing exactly when your mood change happens, as Arthur did, is your starting point. That change is the signpost that tells you: now it's time to gain some control over your feelings (you'll then use the techniques in this chapter as your toolkit).

Worried thoughts

Worried thoughts can race out of control, feel muddled, or perhaps just pop into your mind unexpectedly. Some people hear the same phrase or see the same image again and again, like it's on a loop. Mostly, worried thoughts tend to focus on things that could go wrong. They also often go hand in hand with thoughts such as 'I'll never cope' or 'I can't do this'. All this can make you feel distracted, and powerless.

> The first thing to know is: *thoughts aren't facts*.
>
> A worried thought is just your interpretation:
> *it is NOT a fact*.

For instance, after a social event you might think: 'I really liked meeting that group of people, but I was too quiet and dull – they'll never ask me back'. This feels like a fact. It isn't. It's just your particular 'take' on what happened. In reality, maybe no one will call, or maybe someone will. You can't know for sure either way.

Worried thoughts aren't usually fair and balanced. They are usually weighted in favour of bad things – problems or possible disasters. Usually, when thinking worried thoughts, you also underestimate your ability to cope if bad things did happen.

Use this chapter as a toolkit to help you identify your worried thoughts and replace them with more realistic and balanced ones.

Tackling thought traps

When you're worrying your mind plays tricks on you. It's almost as if your mind wants to keep you feeling wound up. It leads you into 'thought traps' that can be really destructive.

You need to become your own 'thought detective'. This is a very powerful thing. People often say that when they really examine their thought patterns, they can't believe how critical, hard and judgemental they are with themselves.

If you learn to identify exactly what you think when you're worried (your 'thought traps'), then you'll quickly notice just how unbalanced and harsh these thoughts can be.

Nobody is suggesting, by the way, that your thoughts are unbalanced all the time. You might be the most sane, reasonable human being on earth, but when we worry our thoughts do get skewed.

COMMON WORRY THOUGHT TRAPS

1. **Mind reading** (making judgements about what other people are thinking): 'The GP looked worried – she's saying my cough is viral, but she's just trying to protect me, she thinks it is more serious than she is letting on.'

2. **Fortune telling** (predicting the future): 'I can't cope. I'll never work again!'

3. **Thinking the worst** (jumping to the conclusion of the worst outcome without recognising other possibilities): 'If my cancer comes back I won't cope. My wife will leave me and I'll have to face it all alone' or 'My back is sore; it must be a sign the cancer has come back.'

4. **Labelling yourself**: 'I'm so ungrateful. Everyone else gets on with their lives after cancer; I'm just weak.'

5. **If . . . then thinking**: 'If the test results don't come through today . . . then it must be bad news.'

6. **Shoulds and oughts** (unrealistic demands or expectations about yourself): 'I shouldn't feel so upset and stressed.

I've done the hard bit, I ought to be enjoying myself and making the most of this valuable time.'

7. **Selective thinking** (you only remember the bad bits of a situation – you 'forget' about the better bits): 'I'm useless at talking to the consultant about what I need' (but you 'forget' that you actually found ways to communicate with the nurse on the team . . .).

EXERCISE

Keep an anxiety diary

Keeping an anxiety diary will help you to understand the following:

- What makes me worry?
- How do I feel when I get worried?
- What am I saying to myself when I worry?
- What do I tend to do when worried?

Then you can tackle all these things in a way that's really going to work – **for you**.

How to keep an anxiety diary

1. Towards the end of your day, perhaps after your evening meal, take five or ten minutes to review your day.

2. Think back to any incidents in the day that made you worry or feel anxious – write them down.

3. Use a worry scale – see below – to rate the level of worry you felt in each situation.

4. Once you've done steps 1 to 3 for one week the next stage is to understand more about how that feeling works, for you. Jot down the following:

   • What did I feel when the worry hit me? (Slight worry, fear, panic?)

   • What situation was I in? (Where was I? What was happening?)

   • What did I think? (What words started going round my mind?)

   • How did my body feel?

   • What did I do? (What I did to tackle – or avoid – it.)

5. Do step 4 for a week. It will then be time to move on to the 'thought taming' exercise on pages 23–5.

6. Keep your anxiety diary and thought taming exercise going for a month (it's fine if you miss the odd day; no one says you have to be perfect). Looking back through your diary can motivate you: day to day it can be hard to pinpoint changes but over time you'll see you're worrying less.

Your worry scale

• Use a scale from 1 to 10 where 1 is no worries at all and 10 is the most extreme worry.

• Identify a moment when you were worried (what 'set you off'?). Now try to pinpoint, using your scale, how worried you felt. Give that worry a rating from 1 to 10.

• A worry scale will help you to notice when you are getting less anxious over time – you'll notice, for instance, that a worry that was originally an 8 on your scale has become a 6 or even a 5 as you learn to cope better with it.

What now?

Having kept your anxiety diary for a month, it is then up to you, whether you like having a structure to follow and want to keep writing your diary, or if you want to stop. You can always go back to it if you find yourself going through another patch of worrying.

TIP▶

A PERMANENT RECORD

An appointments diary or calendar (or an electronic version such as a Blackberry or iPhone) is useful for this exercise: you can keep a permanent record as you jot down each worry, and its rating.

EXAMPLE

Anxiety diary: Arthur, 71, bowel cancer survivor

INCIDENT: Hearing that Bobby Robson died

WORRY RATING: 8

- **What did I feel?** Sad, worried, fretful, frightened.

- **What was the situation?** Listening to the radio, news item came on.

- **What did I think?** He was so fit and talented, he was such a good person; it is not fair; cancer is so cruel. If it can kill someone like Bobby who must have had the best possible treatment, money no option, then it's bound to kill me –

the doctors say it has gone but I know it will come back to get me.

- **How did my body feel?** Hot, tense, light-headed.

- **What did I do next?** Turned the radio off, got restless, couldn't concentrate, stopped putting photos in album, did the washing up, rearranged bookshelves.

Now try this

Have a look at Arthur's anxiety diary. See if you can spot his thought traps.

- Fortune telling: 'It will come back.'

- Thinking the worst: 'It will kill me.'

- 'If . . . then' thinking: 'If it can kill Bobby then it will kill me.'

You need to become skilled at spotting your own thought traps. With practice, you'll learn to:

- identify the worry thought (yes, even the most worrying ones)

- notice your thought traps

- question and challenge them.

Scary thoughts and why they are OK

It is often very hard to acknowledge your big fears, even to yourself. Many cancer survivors worry that if they think about the bad stuff – including the cancer coming back – then it might happen. This is totally understandable. It's virtually impossible to open a magazine or newspaper without some story cropping up about how positive thinking helped some-one or other to beat cancer.

The thing is, these are just stories – nothing more. Positive thinking is great, and can be useful in helping you to cope better, but it doesn't make the slightest difference to cancer outcomes. Solid scientific research has not found any link between worry about cancer and cancer outcomes.

> Thinking something bad will not make it happen.

If (or when) you find yourself thinking 'I just can't cope. I'm terrified. I know my cancer is going to come back', remind yourself that these thoughts are normal, and they will **not make your cancer come back.**

There is, on the other hand, plenty of scientific evidence to show that learning how to think in a more balanced, realistic, non-panicky way can boost your mood, coping abilities and hugely improve your quality of life. This is why it's worth giving these strategies a go. In fact, that's the whole point of this book.

COPING STRATEGY

Thought taming

After having kept your anxiety diary for two weeks you're going to learn how to manage – and get out of – your thought traps.

To begin with try to tame **one thought** each day for at least a week.

As you get more skilled at taming your thoughts you'll find that you can 'catch' them before they take hold. You will start answering your own worrying thoughts as they happen. Before you know it, you're starting to think in a much more balanced – and much less worried – way.

How to tame your thoughts

1. From your anxiety diary pick one anxious thought you have had during the day.

2. On the left-hand side of your paper write down the actual words that were running through your mind.

3. Now, look back at the thought traps listed above. Have you fallen into any?

4. Ask yourself the following questions about that thought:

- Am I exaggerating any problems or risks?

- What if the thing I'm scared of really did happen? It is difficult to face this question. But if you can, you'll start to think about what you would actually do if it did happen. Surprisingly, just thinking about this reduces the fear.

- What else am I dealing with right now? Am I actually doing quite well, given all the challenges I'm facing and what I've been through?

5. Write the answers to these questions down on the right-hand side of your paper. Now, see if you can come up with more helpful thoughts on the right-hand side, than worrying thoughts on the left-hand side.

And there you have it in a nutshell: more balanced thinking.

TIP▶

'HOLD ON . . .'

If all this debating with yourself seems a bit much at first – and it can be quite a challenge – see if you can catch your thoughts by saying just two words to yourself 'hold on . . .'

'Hold on . . .' will kick off a great new habit: stopping your thought from taking hold, and automatically questioning it. For example, if you're in a 'labelling' thought trap ('I'm pathetic, I never cope with anything'), saying 'Hold on . . .' immediately makes you stop to think: 'Hold on . . . am I really that pathetic? Aren't there some things I've coped with quite well recently?'

But I hate writing

Try not to be put off by all this writing. Writing down thoughts and feelings won't make them disappear but writing does have the useful effect of getting a thought out of your head – and this can be a big relief.

Remember, the writing is just for you: forget about spelling/ handwriting/typing – you're the only one who needs to be able to read it, there's no teacher/boss breathing down your neck here. If writing has never been your thing, and never will be, you can still do all of the exercises suggested in this book just in your mind.

TIP▶

DON'T EXPECT MIRACLES

Changing the way you think takes practice and time. At first, thought taming might feel artificial. You probably won't *believe* the alternative thoughts that you come up with. But when you've done this each day for a week or two you'll get to know the patterns and traps you tend to fall into. And you'll notice that you no longer automatically accept your first thought, but instead you 'catch it' and start to question it.

COPING STRATEGY

'Mindfulness'

Sometimes, you'll have a worrying thought, but you just won't feel like engaging in a debate with yourself, or writing stuff down. At times like this a technique known as mindfulness is a great tool. It takes practice, but it can work wonders. (See Chapter 8: Relax, for more on mindfulness.)

How to do it

Instead of pushing a worrying thought away, or even examining or challenging it, you are going to simply acknowledge that thought. You're not going to judge it. You're just going to watch it go through your head.

When a worrying thought pops into your head try this strategy.

- **Spot it**: It has appeared in your mind.

- **Don't judge it**: There's no need to say 'What a bad, horrible thought'. It's just a thought.

- **Take a moment to think about where you are right here and now**: Use all of your senses. Again, don't judge anything. Just observe yourself. Try to notice things like:
  - the pattern of your breathing
  - background noises
  - the feel of your clothes on your body
  - the position of your body
  - where your feet touch the ground or your back is leaning into the chair
  - how your tongue lies in your mouth
  - any smells wafting over you.

- **Be curious**: Watch your worrying thought, and notice what happens to it, if new thoughts come in to take its place, if it hangs around or disappears.

Mindfulness really can help worries to feel less threatening. The thoughts just come and go. You watch them, but you don't get involved. **They're just thoughts**.

Worried behaviour

When you are worried you behave differently. Sometimes the change is dramatic – shouting, being irrational, tearful or restless. But at other times the behaviour change is so subtle you hardly notice you're doing it. Understanding how, exactly, worry changes your behaviour is an important step towards freeing yourself from anxiety – and getting on with living.

Here are just a few ways in which worries can change your behaviour:

- restlessness – getting up and down, not being able to settle
- difficulty concentrating
- impulsiveness
- impatience
- keeping 'on the go'
- not wanting to stop/slow down/relax
- sleep problems
- needing reassurance from others
- avoiding frightening situations.

Avoidance and why it won't work

You could, of course, just try to avoid or distract yourself from all the things that worry you. This might work OK in the short term. But in the long term it will fail.

Distraction and avoidance can keep a worry going for longer – and even make it worse. If you try to avoid something, you can become quite restricted in how you behave;

your anxieties start dominating your life. This can get exhausting. When you do slow down – and you have to eventually – those worries bounce right back at you.

It's completely reasonable to want to protect yourself – whether your worries are mild or severe. The problem is that human beings are just not very good at suppressing worrying thoughts. In fact, our brains are programmed to look at any given threat from all angles – until we are sure it's gone away. So, when you push a scary thought away, or try to avoid something that worries you, you're only putting the anxiety on hold. It's going to come back. Often it will come back bigger and more worrying than before.

CASE STUDY

Bill, 49, testicular cancer survivor, part 2

Coping with worried behaviour

Bill thought of simple ways to manage his worries in the run up to his annual check-up appointment – a kind of 'worry management strategy'. He decided to:

- *Prepare himself and his family each year, using the clinic appointment letter as a trigger.*

- *Explain to his family that he might be on edge for a bit.*

- *Tell them things they could do to help him, for instance, not asking him why he was so quiet.*

- *Sit down and review the past year, writing down a list of any episodes of ill health or odd physical sensations, as well as times when he felt really well, or any physical successes or achievements, such as joining the local rugby team.*

- *Prepare questions for the medical team, consider what he wants to get from the check-up.*

→

Bill also thought about what helps him when he feels anxious. He realised:

- He finds it easier to cope if he recognises his worried thoughts and gives himself some time to think about the thought traps he is falling into and how to get out of them.

- Exercise helps him to tackle his 'worried body', so he decided to walk the dog in the morning, and do some press-ups before dinner.

Bill's check-up was all good, just as it had been for the previous four years. A few days afterwards, Bill took time to look back over the previous couple of weeks. He noted which of his strategies had turned out to be helpful and which hadn't – and made a few notes. These notes will help him cope even better next year.

Managing your worried behaviour isn't instant. It takes thought and focus – as Bill's approach shows. But it's worth it. Bill felt far more in control both in the run up to his appointment and during it. He is now far less afraid of the fear itself. He still worries a bit, of course, but he knows that he's coping much better – and this is a huge reassurance.

EXERCISE

Pink elephants

Our brains don't respond well when we tell them not to think about something. Try this and you'll see: sit quietly, with your eyes closed. Now, think about absolutely anything except pink elephants.

What did you think about? Chances are that big, hefty pink creatures with trunks featured heavily.

Telling yourself not to think something puts you under enormous pressure to **think it**. You may manage it briefly, but not for long. Those pink elephants are going to rear their trunks at some point whether you like it or not. But if you learn to tame them, you can stop them rampaging through your mind, tearing everything up and leaving a total mess behind.

CASE STUDY

Ally, 64, breast cancer survivor

Facing pink elephants

Ally's huge fear was that her cancer would come back. She did everything she could to avoid thinking about this – filling her time with distractions and tasks – but it wasn't working. However much she tried to avoid thinking about the cancer returning, the thoughts would bounce back at her later – usually at night – and were terrifying when they did.

So, I suggested that she set up a worry time every evening when she would let herself think about what was worrying her and write her anxiety diary. By doing this she found she was gradually able to think through her worst fear. She actually began to work out what she would do if the cancer did come back. Ally discovered that by facing her horrible 'pink elephant', it actually lost some, though obviously not all, of its power to frighten her. She also realised that she was not actually thinking anything new or extra scary. She was not 'opening the floodgates'. She'd had all the thoughts before; it was just that she'd tried to ignore them. Keeping her diary time very well contained really helped

→

Ally to feel she was in control (she set an alarm clock for ten minutes). As soon as the alarm went off, she thought about an achievement from her day, and then she'd throw herself into something she enjoyed – usually cooking the evening meal.

'It does still scare me sometimes,' she told me at our last session. 'But I'm not preoccupied by it like I was – I feel like I'm more in control, I can face it and I know what to do. It's a huge step forward.'

How to manage your worried behaviour

You have to find a way to face the things that worry you, and change your behaviour when you're worried. The way to do this is **gradually, step by step**.

Anxiety follows a pattern. In a scary situation, our level of anxiety:

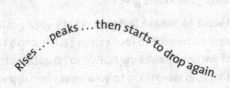

Rises...peaks...then starts to drop again.

You might think that you'll just get more and more panicky if you force yourself to face something you really want to avoid. But if you are brave enough to stay with that anxiety, you'll find that it starts to get less intense. This may all sound alarming. But if you take it slowly, in little steps, it needn't be. In fact, you'll find that changing your behaviour makes you feel much more free.

The key is to start small. Think about someone who is afraid of heights: you're not going to drag them up the London Eye on the first day of 'facing their fear' and force them to look down. Instead, the first step might be to encourage them to stand on a chair in their living room.

EXERCISE

Building your ladder

How to do it

Your anxiety diary (see pages 19–21) will have helped you to understand your worried behaviour: what you tend to do when something sets your worries off (avoidance, distraction, outbursts, tears, panic etc.).

Now, it's time to change that behaviour for the better. Try to work out answers to the following questions.

- **What behaviour do I need to change?** For instance, do you avoid going past your hospital (see Sarah's case study, pages 33–5)? Do you switch off the radio, like Arthur, if something about cancer comes on? Do you shout at your partner? Plough yourself into work? Stick on your trainers and run until your knees give out?

- **How do I want to behave instead?** What's your goal? What do you want to be able to face calmly? (Listen to a radio broadcast without panicking? Drive to hospital without going into a cold sweat? Go to your next check-up without thinking terrifying thoughts?)

- **Now, build your ladder.** You need a step-by-step plan that will take you gradually towards your ultimate goal. Each step should feel manageable. Write your plan down. Bear in mind that it may take you several weeks or longer to get to your goal.

- **Take your first step.** Each step may take days to complete – give it time. Repeat each step until it no longer makes you feel worried. Only then do you move on to the next step.

- **Reward your efforts.** It is incredibly important to recognise and give yourself credit for each step you take up your ladder. If you just focus on the big goal you might think 'I'll never get there'. But each step is important in its own right.

CASE STUDY

Sarah, 50, colon cancer survivor

Managing worried behaviour

Sarah is a married mother of two teenage boys, working full time as an accountant. She was diagnosed with colon cancer three years ago, and had surgery, chemotherapy and radiotherapy.

Sarah responded with 'fighting spirit' to her diagnosis and treatment, was back at work a month after surgery, and combined work and chemotherapy. All her scans and tests were clear and she was followed up by her medical team once every six months. Unfortunately Sarah then found herself overwhelmed by worries about her future.

Her 'symptoms', when worrying, were powerful: a racing heart, fast breathing, hot flushes, thoughts of not being able to cope, not being the person she was before her cancer, not being able to stop thoughts about cancer racing around her head.

She developed complicated ways of 'avoiding' setting off her scary thoughts. She began to drive the long route to work to avoid going past the hospital. She would turn off the radio or TV if a cancer article, programme or advert came on. At home, if a scary thought popped into her head, she'd leap up and clean the house.

→

But she was feeling more and more worried, rather than less. She was ashamed of her worrying – and exhausted. That's when her GP referred her to me.

Sarah used many of the strategies discussed in this chapter to cope with her worries. She kept an anxiety diary, she gave herself worry time, she tamed her thoughts (and recognised that thinking something does not make it happen); she managed her body symptoms using slow breathing, and carrying a bottle of cold water to cool herself down. She also changed her behaviour by facing her biggest fear – the hospital.

Sarah's ladder

My goal: To go right into the hospital without feeling panicky and scared.

Step 1: Drive to a street that leads up to the hospital where I can park but not actually see the hospital.

Step 2: Drive to the street and park where I can see the hospital.

Step 3: Drive past the hospital and park just beyond it with the hospital still in full view.

Step 4: Park in the hospital car park.

Step 5: Park in the car park, go into the hospital coffee shop and walk past the ward where I had much of my treatment.

Sarah used her coping methods as she tackled each step. She'd say encouraging things to herself, too: 'I can do this' and 'This is going to help me'. She repeated each step every day until it no longer made her feel unpleasantly worried. Steps 1 and 2 took five days each. Steps 3, 4 and 5 each took her three to four days to feel comfortable with.

→

Rewarding her efforts

Sarah also came up with a list of 'rewards' to mark each step: watching a DVD with her husband, having a bubble bath, finding time to read a new book, having a family outing at the weekend, ordering a takeaway. By the time we'd finished working together, she told me: 'I'm no longer constantly on the go, afraid to sit still or stop for a second in case thoughts of cancer pop into my head. And my drive to work is much shorter!'

Sometimes she was still worried, of course. She'd been back to the consultant when she felt some pain in her gut. But amazingly, she'd been able to drive herself to that appointment and felt that she got more out of the talk with the consultant, because she wasn't so worried by the surroundings. Sarah's fears have not disappeared completely, but they no longer control her or her family.

Worried bodies

When you are worried or stressed, it shows on your body. 'Worry symptoms' can be mild or extreme, but are never fun.

When you are worried, you may experience:

- racing heart
- rapid breathing
- butterflies in the stomach
- sweating
- blushing
- frequent trips to the loo
- muscle tension

- light-headedness
- restlessness and jitters.

Learning to recognise your worry symptoms clearly will help you, first of all, to reassure yourself that there isn't something physically wrong with you – you aren't about to drop down dead of a heart attack, and you aren't going mad. This will immediately take your worry down a notch. You can then learn tricks to reduce the unpleasant physical feelings. Again, this is going to reduce the worry itself and make you feel much more calm and in control in general.

How to manage your worried body

When you're worried, stressed or nervous you've sensed a 'threat'. Your body goes on high alert: adrenaline starts pumping through your veins, getting you ready to run away or fight that threat (the 'fight–flight' response). Of course, when it comes to post-cancer worries, there is nothing to flee from – or to fight. This means that your body is left with pent-up energy, and nowhere for it to go.

This explains why:

- your muscles feel tight and tense
- your heart beats faster
- you breathe faster
- you feel hot, sweaty or light-headed.

TIP▶

PANIC ATTACKS

Panic attacks are an extreme version of the worried body. A panic attack can leave you thinking 'I am going to collapse' or 'I can't breathe'. If you do have a panic attack you need to release this physical tension quickly (starting with number 1 on the list below). You also need to reassure yourself that although what you're feeling is horrible, it isn't dangerous or life-threatening, and you can control it. The strategies listed here all help with panic attacks, as well as other worries and fretful situations.

Five ways to cope with your worried body:

1. **Slow your breathing down**. A good strategy is to get your 'out breath' to last for longer than your 'in breath'. Say to yourself as you breathe in: 'In 1, 2, 3'. Then hold your breath and count to 2 or 3. Then, as you breathe out, say to yourself: 'Out 1, 2, 3, 4, 5'. Keep doing this until you feel more relaxed. Also try: The 'straws, balloons and feathers' trick. If counting doesn't work for you try imagining, as you breathe out, that you are blowing through a straw, blowing up a balloon or keeping a feather floating up in the air. All three of these images encourage you to purse your lips and, if your lips are pursed, you can't breathe out too fast.

2. **Get moving**. You don't have to start jogging (though that kind of exercise works wonders if you are up to it). A walk round the block, or even just a change of position or some gentle stretching – anything you can manage – will help burn off some of that pent-up adrenaline. Also try: climbing some stairs, doing some star jumps, jogging on the spot, going for a walk in the park, kicking a football in the garden.

3. **Get a gadget**. Check out some of the stress reliever gadgets you can buy these days: carrying one of those squashy balls in your bag or using a mini back massager can help calm your body down.

4. **Cool down**. If you get hot when you worry, just splashing some water on your face can help. Also try: keeping a bottle

of cold water with you to drink or splash, using wet wipes over your face or hands, or carry one of those little hand-held battery operated fans people use in summer.

5. **Relaxation techniques**. Relax, dammit! Of course, barking at yourself to calm down won't work. In fact, pressurising yourself to relax can make you even more wound up. But there are many easy relaxation techniques that don't necessarily involve hours of meditating in silent, dark rooms (see Chapter 8: Relax). Relaxation is a skill, though. Learning and practising it when you are not in a total tizzy is a very sensible starting point for coping with worries generally.

TIP ▶

SLOW DOWN AND PLAN

OK, so you may have noticed what seems like a mixed message: to manage your worried body you need to get moving (see page 37). But, if you get too active, and start distracting yourself all the time, or avoiding your fears by throwing yourself into tasks then you are just stacking up problems for later. This can be a bit of a dilemma. The key is to find a balance between burning off the physical effects of your pent-up worries, and calmly looking at the worries themselves. So, when you feel anxious, you could try to do something active that allows you to look at and question your worrying thoughts at the same time: for instance, going for a walk or swim, or doing some gardening.

It can also help to plan, in advance, what you will do when you feel anxious (for example 'I will take a ten-minute walk', 'I will prune the roses for five minutes', 'I will go for a twenty-minute swim'). Planning, with time limits, can stop you feeling out of control and going too far and just distracting yourself with activity when your worries kick in.

Coping with the fear that cancer will come back

For most people, coping with the fear that cancer will come back is the greatest challenge of all when treatment ends.

'Every time I get tired, lose a pound in weight, or feel a lump in my neck I think the cancer is back,' says Clare, 23, lymphoma survivor.

The fear brings its 'symptoms' along with it: the racing, intrusive, upsetting thoughts; the worry, frustration, nervousness; the body symptoms – muscle tension, fast heartbeat, quick breathing, nausea; and the behaviour changes – avoidance, doing too much, finding it hard to concentrate, being irritable, needing reassurance, feeling restless.

After cancer it is completely natural to assume the worst. You feel a twinge of pain somewhere – you immediately think, 'It's a sign that the disease has spread'. You've had to face unexplained symptoms before. You may have tried to reassure yourself then, and look what happened: cancer.

TIP▶

GET ADVICE AND SUPPORT FROM THE EXPERTS

There is no way that you're going to be able to face odd physical feelings without some degree of worry or panic. No Survivor's Companion book – or person – is going to stop this from happening. It's normal, natural and understandable. It takes time, and also experience, to understand how you might feel when treatment has finished. But in the early stages, you just aren't experienced in the physical after-effects of cancer. You are right not to ignore new physical sensations. It is therefore perfectly reasonable to get information or advice from your medical team. This is an essential part of managing the health of your body and your mind after cancer.

CASE STUDY

Clare, 23, lymphoma survivor

Clare's worry plan

I first met Clare during her treatment for lymphoma when she had a difficult hospital admission. She asked to see me again after her discharge from treatment because she was very worried about her physical sensations but also really worried that she was 'bothering the medical team too much: they must think I am a total hypochondriac'.

Together, we came up with a worry management plan.

- **Information gathering**: First, Clare got detailed information from her haematology team about what signs they would want to check out. Now she knew when to contact them. The consultant reassured her that he expected her to want some extra appointments between their regular follow ups – she'd be learning about her body and would need information and advice. He'd expect her to need fewer of these appointments as time went on.

- **Communication**: Clare talked to her clinical nurse specialist about how worried she was about being a hypochondriac. The nurse said she'd much rather hear from Clare than think of her suffering at home on her own. They agreed that Clare could email her nurse with any questions or concerns. (This felt more comfortable and less intrusive for Clare and the nurse than telephoning.) She also talked to her GP about her fears of unexplained physical sensations. The very understanding and helpful GP told Clare that for at least the first year after treatment she had a 'hypochondria licence' and could consult her whenever she wanted. This was far better than missing something. Like the haematology team Clare's GP also

→

suggested that Clare would need less reassurance as time went by.

- **Thought taming**: Clare then started learning that instead of accepting her first thought as a fact ('The tiredness and lump means the illness is back'), she could question it. She asked herself about other possible explanations for her symptoms. For instance, she learned from her consultant and her GP that her lymph nodes and glands would swell in response to any viral or bacterial infection; she learned that her weight fluctuated within a range of a few pounds according to her diet, exercise levels and menstrual cycle; and her tiredness levels had a lot to do with work demands. Clare also faced her 'What if it did come back?' thought. She realised that she'd cope with lymphoma second time round in the same way that she had done first time. It would be incredibly difficult but she had found inner resources she did not know she had last time. She'd used support from family, friends and medical staff. She'd bonded with other patients. She'd used her yoga skills. All those resources would still be there if her cancer came back – plus she knows now that she has greater resilience than she ever thought possible. Clare also looked at the things she was saying to herself – she tried to talk to herself in a kinder way, as if talking to a good friend. She used the 'hold on' strategy whenever she found that she was being harsh or critical of herself and this took a lot of pressure off.

- **Other coping strategies**: Clare also combined some relaxation strategies, regular exercise (her yoga), mindfulness techniques and rewards to help her to feel better.

She told me in our last session: 'When I feel something new I am not sure I will ever be able to stop my first thought being that it is the lymphoma back. But what I can do now is stop beating myself up about it. I can use my experience to find other

➡

> *possible explanations and decide if I need to get medical advice or not.' Clare admitted that this took a lot of work, but she felt it had paid off. She was far less worried. She felt she was getting her life back.*

Be good to yourself

Worrying can be exhausting and unpleasant. You really need to give yourself a break sometimes. Imagine if you were talking to a good friend about this. You might say to them, 'Hey, you need to look after yourself, find a way to feel better, you've been through so much.' So, why be harder on yourself than you would be on a friend?

Have a think about things that you find soothing – maybe talk to your family about it, come up with a list. Whatever makes you feel good – a long hot bubble bath, a computer game, an evening with friends, listening to music, playing with the dog, a game of darts – is important.

Now, reward yourself at least once a week with something from your list. Plan for this, and follow it through. If you're tempted to think this sort of thing is self-indulgent, don't: lots of scientific studies show that rewards or 'soothing yourself' are vital when you are trying to change your thoughts and behaviour. They make a huge difference to your chances of success here. So don't sell yourself short.

What now?

Whether your brand of worry is mild or really problematic, the bottom line is that it is a totally normal side effect of cancer survival. But if you ignore your anxieties – or let them rule you – then you are never going to fully feel good about your post-cancer life.

Some of the techniques in this chapter will sound difficult, confusing, maybe even frightening, or too time-consuming. The thing is that they are all proven methods, backed up by reliable scientific research. They're not silly, touchy-feely tricks made up by a couple of authors with too much time on their hands. These psychological methods and techniques have helped thousands of people, just like you, to cope much, much better after cancer. And they get easier, the more you do them. Believe it or not, they will become second nature if you practise.

Conquering your worries – getting them under control – frees you up to do other things. It lets you get on with your life. You can start this any time: so how about now?

Family, friends and carers: How you can help with worries

One thing to remember above all: worry is a **normal** part of life after cancer.

It can be incredibly difficult to watch someone you care about feeling worried and unsettled. You might feel worried too. Or frustrated. Or stressed out. Or all of the above. But your loved one may just need to go through this before they can feel better. It's important to know that you can't 'make them feel better'. However, there are certainly things you can do to help them get through this.

Helping a worrier: Dos and don'ts

- **Don't say** 'You mustn't think like that!' or 'Just put it out of your mind'. Read this chapter's section on pink elephants (see pages 29–30) for a full explanation of why this isn't a good thing to say. Instead:
- **Do** try to be a listening ear. Let them talk.

- **Don't** dismiss their fears or worries ('That's just silly' or 'You aren't going to get anywhere if you keep panicking'). Instead:

- **Do** try to accept that even if the worries seem crazy or pointless to you, it's something they are genuinely feeling and wrestling with.

- **Don't** try to solve or answer their problems ('You should just … ') or reassure them ('That's not going to happen'). You don't need to have the answers – in fact, trying to answer and reassure a person in this situation may not be helpful at all. Instead:

- **Do** listen (see above) and encourage them to think through 'What if …?' (What if that 'worst case scenario' really happened?), rather than trying to push these thoughts away. Helping them to face and talk through their fears can be invaluable.

- **Don't** let all this talking dominate your life. Worry and fear can – and often do – become repetitive and intrusive. If you find that you're frequently going over the same material, and you're feeling overwhelmed or fed up with this, then talk can actually become counterproductive. Instead:

- **Do** introduce some structured daily (or weekly, or every other day – whatever suits you) 'talk time' (see pages 148–50). Then you can say: 'This is not our talk time; let's talk about this properly at XX p.m.'

- **Don't** not try to force them to talk. Some people who are anxious just don't want to talk. Instead:

- **Do** let them know you are available any time if they do need to talk.

Helping with things in this chapter

You can also help with the strategies right here in this book:

• Read this chapter carefully so you understand more about the anxiety and how to tackle it.

• Show an interest in their efforts.

• Offer your support – recognise that it can be hard to tackle worries and anxiety, listen when they are complaining that 'it's impossible'.

• Celebrate their successes and point out any positive changes you see as a result of their efforts, however small.

Three good places to start:

1. **Avoidance**: You may be able to offer practical help here (see pages 27–8). You can offer to help them draw up the 'worry ladder' (pages 32–3) and may be able to help them achieve certain steps on the way to their goal. But if you do this, also be aware of the dos and don'ts above. Your urge may be to protect, shield and reassure them – you want to make all these awful worries vanish. But you can't really do that. Remember: a person needs to face a fear in order to overcome it.

2. **Relaxation**: Learn some relaxation exercises to do together to tackle anxiety and tension. It can be motivating to have someone learn alongside you, and – given the pressure and stress you are (and have been) under – you will undoubtedly benefit from these techniques too.

3. **Exercise**: Encourage them and possibly even go with them as they build up a gradual exercise programme as a way to tackle their body tension and stress. An 'exercise buddy' is a priceless accessory when you're trying to motivate your-self – and, as above, it can really help you to unwind and deal with the pressure you're under too.

CHAPTER TWO

DEPRESSION AND LOW MOOD

> I thought this would be it, the moment when I could let go of all the pressure and stress and get back to enjoying my life. But if anything I feel less happy now than I ever have before. Surely it's not meant to be like this? I should be happy.

GERRY, 70, KIDNEY CANCER SURVIVOR

Low mood – or even depression – is one of the most common side effects of cancer.

Sometimes this feeling kicks in almost as soon as treatment ends, but it might also hit you months or even years later. There are many reasons why your mood might plummet after treatment, but the basic summary is simple: you've been through a very tough experience (physically and emotionally) and it takes time to recover.

You've had to adjust to some serious changes in your life – both during treatment and now that it's over. You've faced all sorts of losses, and you need time to grieve for these. Your coping abilities – both physical and mental – have been stretched to the limit (and beyond). You need time to get your strength back.

If you feel depressed – 'down', 'low', 'miserable' – you are not mentally ill, you are not going mad, you are not ungrateful or a wimp and you do not automatically require professional help (though you may find this very useful). You are just feeling sad. You're finding a way to make sense of everything that has happened to you. You may be in a difficult place, but you will adjust. This chapter will give you ways to do this.

What is depression?

It might sound like an obvious question, but, in fact, it can be hard to pin down exactly what depression is. Absolutely everyone feels low from time to time. But when does 'low' turn into 'depressed'? Unlike cancer, there's no scan, blood or other physical test that will confirm a diagnosis of depression. It is just a cluster of 'symptoms' – some in your body, some in your behaviour and some in your thoughts – that together make you feel different, unhappy and stuck.

In fact, scientists have tried very hard to pinpoint exactly how to diagnose depression. After endless elaborate scientific research studies, this is what they've come up with: one of the most effective ways to diagnose depression is simply to ask the person, 'Are you depressed?'

If you'd like more information before you answer, then the list below might help you. It outlines some general features of depression. Everyone experiences one or two of these from time to time. But, as a rough guide, if you find that you have at least five of the symptoms below, and they last a minimum of two weeks, then you may be showing signs of depression. But the chances are that if you are depressed, you already know it.

SYMPTOMS OF DEPRESSION

- Sadness, most of the time
- Crying
- Thinking negative things about yourself, the world and the future
- Losing interest in other people
- Not enjoying activities that you used to enjoy
- Feeling lethargic and lacking motivation
- Appetite changes
- Sleep difficulties
- Feeling helpless or hopeless
- Feeling that you've lost self-esteem or self-confidence
- Blaming or disliking yourself
- Feeling guilty
- Feeling irritable
- Withdrawing from other people
- Having problems concentrating
- Not looking after yourself, for example paying less attention to your appearance, personal hygiene, or using alcohol or drugs too much
- Feeling tired
- Getting aches and pains or muscle tension etc.

The vicious circle of depression

Depression involves thoughts, feelings and behaviour. These influence each other in a circular way, like this:

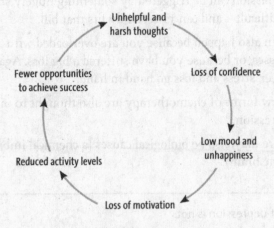

The depression circle

How common is depression?

In general, around one in four or five of us will experience at least one episode of depression in our lifetime. At any one time around 10 per cent of the adult population may be suffering from depression. It can affect people of any age, both men and women. But it probably won't surprise you to learn that when it comes to living with, and beyond, cancer the rates of depression are higher. It can be hard to pin down the exact number of people suffering from depression after cancer but research studies have indicated that between 25 and 40 per cent of people may go through some depression after cancer.

Why does this happen?

The current medical theory is that depression is a combination of life events, biology and genes. It can happen very suddenly or it can build up more gradually. In some cases there is no obvious reason – but clearly, for you as a cancer survivor, this is not the case.

- Depression can be triggered by something hugely stressful or difficult – and cancer certainly fits that bill.

- It can also happen because you are overloaded with stresses, or because you have suffered a big loss. Again, cancer, stress and loss go hand in hand.

- A few forms of chemotherapy are also thought to induce depression.

- There may also be biological causes (a chemical imbalance in the brain).

What depression is **not**:

- It is not a sign of weakness, failure or self-indulgence.

- It is not something that you can just 'snap out of'.

- It is not your fault.

Treatment for depression: Getting out of the jungle

Depression is a bit like a jungle: a dark, frightening, dense and confusing place that's hard to get out of. With help, it is much easier to beat your path through that jungle, than it is if you go it alone. The good news is that depression can be treated. It's therefore a really good idea to talk to someone who knows about depression – a GP, nurse, counsellor or psychologist. They can give you support and advice that will get you through the jungle. There are many treatment methods that work really well.

If you can't stand the idea of putting yet more chemicals into your body, don't despair: many really good treatments don't involve medication at all.

Many people with depression will put it behind them if they get information, support and some practical and tested coping strategies.

Possible paths out of your depression jungle

- **Time, information and reassurance**: Sympathetic friends or family and the simple passing of time are enough to get some people through this difficult adjustment. But sometimes people do need more than this.

- **Tackling depressed behaviour**: Some people respond well to practical strategies that help them to get back to being more active; doing what they need – and want – to do.

- **Tackling depressed thoughts**: Other people find it helpful to examine their thought processes. They learn to identify the tricks of the mind that keep them feeling down, to recognise their 'thought traps' and to develop new and more helpful ways of thinking.

- **Medication**: This can be a useful starting point for some people because it can help to lift their mood so they can find the motivation to get back on track (see pages 78–9).

- **A combo**: For most people some combination of the above works best.

'Yeah, right'

When you're depressed, it's hard to believe that anything can possibly change. As you read this, you may have already started thinking, 'Yeah, right, well none of that's going to work on me'. You're not being difficult. You're just feeling depressed, and this way of thinking goes with the territory.

As you progress through this chapter try to catch yourself thinking things like this:

- This will never work.
- I can't do this.
- What good will it do?
- What's the point?
- This is way too simplistic: my life is far more complicated than this.
- I never manage to stick at anything so I won't even bother to start.
- Nothing I try ever works out; this isn't going to be any different.
- I'll start this when I have more energy/support/ motivation.
- It's OK for these authors to write something down in a book, but actually doing it is a completely different kettle of fish.

If the last thought has already hit you, you're actually right. It's way easier to give advice than follow it. Getting out of depression can be incredibly hard. Following some of the advice in this chapter might not banish your depression, but it will start you on the path out of this jungle. And that's a huge step forward.

TIP ▶

PERSEVERE

If all you want to do is to curl up in bed and pull the covers over your head, then it takes incredible strength to get up and try these strategies. The changes will be slow. Sometimes they'll be too subtle even to notice, especially in the early days. But keep going. These strategies are scientifically tried and tested. They do work if you can make yourself do them.

It is also worth reminding yourself that:

Finishing cancer treatment is not just an end point;
it is also a beginning of recovery and rebuilding.

You *will* feel better.

But why am I sad *now*?

Your cancer treatment is over. You're 'supposed' to be happy, relieved – over the moon, even. In fact, many cancer survivors feel the exact opposite.

'I thought that once I got to the end of my treatment and put the cancer behind me, everything would be OK again,' says Jake, 25, skin cancer survivor. 'But I don't feel that the cancer is behind me. Nothing feels right. I know I'm lucky; I know that I should be relieved, maybe even happy, but I'm not. I feel stuck and lost and I don't know how to put things right.'

Jake is one of countless people who discover that the end of treatment is not the 'happy ending' they assumed it would be. Cancer is frightening, stressful and physically exhausting. It disrupts not just your daily life, but also your long-standing plans and ambitions. If you have previously had depression you stand a higher risk of getting depressed again during or after cancer. But depression can hit absolutely anyone after cancer.

There are several reasons for this:

1. Expectations – your own, and other people's.

2. Your body – physical challenges, getting your strength back.

3. Your emotions – getting over the trauma and exhaustion.

The pressure of expectations

'I resolved never to grumble again about little things,' says Vera, 68, eye cancer survivor. 'I vowed to appreciate and enjoy every single day after cancer because every day would be a bonus.'

Often people who are going through cancer treatment make deals with themselves about what they'll do if and when they get the 'all-clear'. 'I told myself, and my wife, that if I got through this I would put the rest of my life to good use', says Keith, 45, leukaemia survivor. 'We talked about how I'd leave my boring, unimportant job in accounts. We'd set up a residential home together to provide a loving and homely atmosphere for elderly people in their twilight years.'

But the pressure 'to make the most of life' can – and often does – backfire. It can feel overwhelming. And this can leave you very confused, lost and low.

How often have you read newspaper articles about 'my second chance at life', where a celebrity puts their cancer experience to brilliant use, fundraising, publicising and supporting other people? These survivors really are doing something amazing. They say that cancer changed their whole life – sometimes even for the better. This is an extraordinary achievement. But it's just that: out of the ordinary.

Most people, after cancer, find their own quiet way of picking up the pieces and carrying on, much as before. But this is actually incredible too: it can be a huge challenge just to get back on track after cancer. Unfortunately these stories don't sell newspapers or make gripping TV shows.

You are also probably well aware, by now, of how terrified

other people are just by the word cancer. This fear changes how people treat you, both during and after your treatment. They want to hear that life after cancer is completely fantastic. They want to know that if you go through hell, you come out on top. This makes it all seem less threatening to them (they know, after all, that they could get cancer one day too).

Until you went through cancer you were probably one of those people. Maybe even now you have some of those hopes and expectations for yourself. But even if you don't put this sort of pressure on yourself, the chances are that other people will do it for you.

'My husband wants to throw a party for me to celebrate the end of my cancer,' says Anila, 52, breast cancer survivor. 'He's so happy and excited but I don't feel that way at all. I don't want to celebrate; I don't feel happy. I feel down and worried. I can't even be bothered to get myself looking presentable when I go out: how on earth would I manage a party?'

Sometimes even healthcare teams can add to this pressure without thinking. Jake, 25, skin cancer survivor (mentioned above) was told by his GP: 'Get yourself back to university, throw yourself into everything that it has to offer. Work hard, play hard and have a great life.'

If only it was that simple.

Your body after treatment

Your body and your mood are linked. And your body has taken a huge hit. You may be scarred and shaken up. You may have lost parts of your body and suffered enormously. You may feel overwhelmed by side effects such as fatigue, mobility difficulties, pain, discomfort or lymphoedema. On top of this, your general level of strength and fitness will probably have dropped.

The Victorians had a concept of 'convalescence'. They

recognised that after a major illness it takes someone time to recover and regain their strength. But over the years – maybe because of the amazing advances in medical treatments – we've somehow lost this valuable idea.

Our attitudes towards our bodies have radically changed. Take childbirth. Nowadays, women are supposed to spring up almost immediately the baby is out. But in days gone by they were given valuable time to rest, recover and adjust.

The same goes for cancer. The expectation these days is that you should be raring to go the moment you are discharged (or even as soon as the time between follow-up appointments is lengthened). Sometimes this can feel overwhelming.

'My boss rang me to ask when I would be going back to work the day I was discharged by my cancer team,' says Shakira, 39, cervical cancer survivor. 'My husband says it is a coincidence but it feels to me like my boss has already forgotten what I have been through. He's pressurising me all over again.'

Your mind and emotions after treatment

It's easy to forget that just by getting through cancer and its treatment, you have achieved something astonishing.

Just for a moment, think about the mental effort it took you to walk into the chemotherapy suite or the hospital waiting room week after week. Think about how much effort it took to put a smile on your face when the kids got home from school, or to chat with your neighbour while battling pain or nausea. This is hard work and you've done it day in day out throughout treatment. It's the mental equivalent of having run a marathon, climbed Ben Nevis, swum the Channel – or all three. No wonder you're exhausted.

'It is almost as if my mind, which has been one of my greatest strengths through my cancer treatment, gave itself permission to collapse,' says David, 64, prostate cancer survivor.

'It feels like my mind's just stopped. It's drained, empty, it's just checked out.'

CASE STUDY

Anila, 52, breast cancer survivor

When Anila's breast cancer treatment ended, she was shocked by how low she felt. She began to think very negative, harsh things about herself. 'I'm pathetic,' she told me at our first session. 'I can't clean the house as well as I once did. Visitors will see how hopeless I am if they come round. I should be able to keep it spotless like I used to. No one will want to come over. I feel so guilty – I'm getting everything wrong. I can't look after my family any more. I'm a failure as a wife and a mother.'

These thoughts were constantly going round Anila's head. She almost didn't notice them, she just accepted them. Gradually, she became more and more withdrawn. By the time she saw me, she'd reached the stage where she'd get out of bed in the morning to see her two teenage children off to school, do a small amount of cleaning, then go back to bed, only getting up again in time to cook dinner.

When I first met Anila, she was treating her thoughts like facts. We talked about how these thoughts were really just her own perspective on a situation – they weren't necessarily accurate (see Chapter 1: Worries).

I also explained that, for some unknown reason the brain works hard to keep us depressed: it lays thought traps for us . When we're depressed, our brains actually make it harder to remember happy or successful events. We focus on small things that have gone wrong rather than the bigger, successful picture. We

→

automatically assume the worst. So, I worked with Anila to identify the 'thought traps' she was falling into, and do something about them.

Anila's depressed thought traps

- *Labelling herself: 'I'm pathetic.'*

- *Mental filtering: As if you're wearing a pair of glasses that filter out what you're actually achieving. 'I can't clean as well as I once did' (here, Anila has 'filtered out' the fact that she's cleaning the house in the first place).*

- *Unrealistic or harsh expectations: 'I should be able to keep it spotless.'*

- *Mind reading: 'Visitors will see how hopeless I am.'*

- *Fortune telling: 'No one will want to come over.'*

- *'All or nothing' thinking: 'I can't keep the house clean; I cannot look after my family any more' (meaning that Anila saw house cleaning as the only way of caring for her family).*

- *Thinking the worst: 'I'm a failure as a wife and mother.'*

By identifying these thought traps, Anila realised that many of her thoughts weren't actually factual or realistic. Now she could do something about them. This was her first step towards lifting herself out of this depression, and moving on.

'I can't go on'

For some people, the depression gets so bad that they start to think they might not want to carry on. These things are incredibly difficult to talk about. They can be frightening for you to say, and alarming for the person you're saying them to.

But thinking you want the suffering to stop, not wanting to wake up, or thinking it's not worth carrying on are all more common than you'd think. Your healthcare team wouldn't be surprised or scared if you told them you were thinking this way.

People often say they feel weak or stupid when they have these thoughts. But if you are thinking these things you're actually very brave – you're carrying on, despite thinking this, and that takes courage.

However, there is a crucial difference between exhausted thoughts ('How much longer can I go on like this?', 'I wish this suffering would end') and the more rare, but active suicidal thoughts, where you actually plan how you'll do it.

If you are having active suicidal thoughts **never ignore them**. You need help, immediately, and help is available. Talk to a member of your medical team, your GP, or call a helpline such as Samaritans (see page 260).

COPING STRATEGY

How to manage depression

Step 1: Recovery time

Instead of telling yourself you shouldn't feel low, try to allow yourself time to feel this way. It's OK – it's normal – to feel like this, after what you've been through. You aren't wallowing. You aren't going to feel this way forever. You don't *want* to feel this way. You're not to blame.

What you actually need is time and space to convalesce. Sadly you can't pack yourself off to a Victorian clinic in the Swiss Alps. But try to think in terms of recovery time. Do try to work out how best to look after yourself while you 'convalesce'.

Why depression won't make the cancer come back

There's this idea (again, it's a huge media and social pressure these days) that you 'should' think positive – that thinking positive will help you stay cancer free. It won't. In fact, feeling low or depressed will **not** raise the risk of your cancer coming back. Numerous major scientific studies back this up. Remember this:

Gloomy, unhappy, anxious thoughts have no effect on cancer cells.

Step 2: Give yourself time to grieve

You have lost a lot because of cancer. Maybe you lost your job, missed out on a promotion; maybe your finances suffered, your fertility was damaged, your pain-free life vanished, your fitness went – or even parts of your body. Maybe you couldn't get to a family wedding, missed your child's first day at school or the chance to be actively involved in your grandchild's first year of life. Perhaps you can't live independently any more, or prune your garden, or do a sport you loved. Above all, you've lost that sense that you're invincible. Of course, logically you knew you weren't superhuman before the cancer hit. But you never really had to face up to that fact. Everyone, post-cancer, has their own list of losses. Most are likely to be long. It's OK to let yourself be sad about this.

EXERCISE

Permission to grieve time

- Go somewhere private where you won't be disturbed (your bedroom, in the bath).

- Put on some sad music if you want.

- Think about your losses.

- Acknowledge how your life has changed.

- Cry if you want to.

- Set a firm time limit on this – fifteen minutes at most. Set an alarm, or get a friend to call you at the end of your grieving time. It can also help to do this just before your favourite TV show or something else that you enjoy: this will help you to move on when your time for being sad is finished.

TIP ▶

DON'T WORRY, IT'S NOT WALLOWING

This exercise isn't going to open a nasty can of worms. You won't be wallowing in self-pity. It won't make you more depressed. And it won't make your cancer come back. It's really just the pink elephants from Chapter 1 again: if you push your sadness and grief away it won't just vanish. It'll pop back up again – probably worse.

Step 3: Live well

There are a lot of practical ways to tackle depression, and many very effective ones involve simple lifestyle changes. Here are the essential ones.

Eat well for energy

These five basic healthy eating tips will help your energy levels and well-being. Always check with your healthcare team as well, in case they have any specific dietary advice for you.

1. **Eat three meals a day**. Don't skip meals and try to eat them at regular intervals: plan and ideally shop in advance so you

have good, nutritious choices. Even if you have a very limited appetite, try to make sure that you have three set mealtimes and that what little you do feel like eating is nutritious. Equally, if your appetite has increased, it is a good idea to plan three healthy and sustaining meals each day: this will help you to control your eating and avoid too much snacking between meals.

2. **Choose whole grains** where possible, rather than white or processed foods.

3. **Go for low-fat** dairy products such as skimmed or semi-skimmed milk and yoghurt.

4. **Eat at least five portions of fruit and vegetables** a day and try to 'eat the rainbow' (by having as many different coloured foods on your plate as you can, such as carrots, red peppers, green leafy veg, bananas). This will give you plenty of 'antioxidants', which boost the immune system and help to protect you from disease.

5. **Eat some 'good fats' daily**. They are found in oily fish such as salmon and mackerel, seeds, walnuts and rapeseed oil. Limit 'bad fats' – these are the 'saturates' that are found in animal products such as butter, cheese and meats as well as in cakes, biscuits and pastries.

TIP ▶

DRINK WELL

- Drink more water! Aim for at least eight tall glasses a day – this can, amazingly, give you more energy, and help your digestion.

- Keep your alcohol intake low (alcohol saps your energy).

- Avoid fizzy drinks or cordials (they contain sugar that will give you a temporary burst, followed by an energy 'crash').

- Fruit juice is fine in moderation – a glass of fresh fruit juice is one of your 'five a day', but remember, even pure fruit juice contains sugars that can give you energy boosts and crashes.
- Cut down on caffeine – in coffee, tea as well as colas – as it will also give you temporary energy bursts followed by dips.

Snacking

You may have been brought up thinking snacks are bad, but in fact, eating the right kind of snack is a good way to keep your blood sugar levels steady. This will help to keep your energy on an even keel (which, in turn, can really help with fatigue and motivation). Obviously, if you snack on things like crisps and Mars Bars you aren't going to do yourself any favours (sugary or fatty snacks will make you more tired – they'll give you a temporary boost, and then your energy will 'crash'). It can help to plan your snacks, just as you plan your meals. Choose foods that provide a steady supply of energy, vitamins and minerals without loading you up with too much fat, sugar or salt.

Here are five healthy snack ideas:

1. A banana and a handful of plain (not roasted or salted) nuts such as Brazil nuts or almonds.
2. Carrot sticks to dip into hummus.
3. A piece of cheese or lean ham and a pear.
4. A bowl of wholegrain cereal with skimmed or semi-skimmed milk.
5. Slice of wholegrain toast with low-fat cheese spread or peanut butter, and a tomato.

TIP►

LIMIT CAFFEINE, ALCOHOL AND (AS IF YOU NEED TELLING) NICOTINE

All three drugs have short-term stress-relieving effects, but overall, too much caffeine is not good for your well-being. Smoking will do major damage, as will too much alcohol.

Grooming and personal hygiene

Try to go back to your old 'grooming' routines: your daily showers, washing your clothes regularly, taking trips to the barber/hairdresser (there are many who are used to working with people after cancer). Go back to any massages, manicures, pedicures you used to enjoy (or start them now, you deserve it!). If you were a clean-shaven man before the cancer and your facial hair is growing, then shave daily. Keeping your body 'groomed' is a vital part of feeling good about yourself.

Get active

Moving around more really is the wonder drug. Recent scientific research shows that regular exercise such as walking is just as good, if not better, than antidepressants for treating people with mild to moderate depression.

When you move more, you build up your physical strength and fitness. This can boost your confidence and self-esteem. Being more active during the day will also help you to relax and sleep better at night. What's more, after a burst of activity your body releases endorphins – the 'feel good' chemicals that lift your mood.

You don't have to suddenly take up kick-boxing (keep in mind the idea of convalescence), but try to build up to about thirty minutes of moderate activity on most days of the week.

Any movement that gets you warm and slightly out of breath counts.

There is clear research evidence that a thirty-minute walk every other day has a significant impact on the mental and physical well-being of cancer survivors.

It is important not to overdo this, particularly at first. You will probably need to pace yourself and build up your activity levels gradually. See Chapter 6: Fatigue for help with how to pace your activity, and always check with your healthcare team that your plans are right for you.

Get moving: Six simple ideas

1. **Make a walk your daily habit.** For instance, take the dog for a walk or set a regular morning walk date with a friend ('walking buddy'). If you can find a green place to walk in – a park or wood or riverside – that's even better.

2. **Build walking into your everyday activities**. Get off the bus two stops early on your way to work, walk instead of drive to the shops, walk round the block for ten minutes in your lunch hour. Also, try to take the stairs whenever you can – you'll be amazed how often you get moving if you avoid lifts and escalators.

3. **Go swimming**. This is another good exercise as it supports the body and so minimises pain and impact. Most local swimming pools offer exercise classes in the pool, which can be great as they tend to be gentle, and virtually anyone can participate, whatever level of physical ability. In summer, you could even try an outdoor pool if you have one locally, to combine the benefits of fresh air and movement.

➡

4. **Join classes or groups**. Don't worry about pump aerobics – try a stretch, Pilates or yoga class (which will have calming benefits too), or maybe a dance class. (Have a word with the class leader before you start so he or she can support you as you set the pace for your activity level and build up your stamina.) There may even be a walking group in your local area. The key here is to find something you enjoy. You may meet people, and become part of a group, which can also help to make you feel happier.

5. **Do some gardening**. Weeding, digging and mowing the lawn all count as moderate activity and get you outside in the fresh air, surrounded by nature – again, a brilliant mood booster.

6. **Do the housework**. Brisk housework such as mopping, vacuuming, dusting and DIY all counts as activity, as does dancing in front of the mirror with your head-phones on.

TIP ▶

GET OUT!

If you can, try to get outside as much as possible and ideally head for green spaces. Nature, even if it's the trees in your local city park, is calming, and uplifting. Just being outside, looking at the trees or feeling the rain on your face and the wind in your hair can boost your mood. Try to really revel in the sensations you feel outdoors – the sound of the wind in the trees, the feel of rain on your face, the warmth of the sun on your arms, the smell of the spring flowers or the cut grass.

Step 4: Monitor your progress

Almost everyone who is low or depressed says, or thinks, 'I'm not coping; I'm not getting anything done'. Low mood and depression change the way you look at life. It's like wearing glasses that filter out the things you actually achieve, leaving your day looking empty, grey and pointless.

Some of the things you achieve each day might seem mundane or trivial to you. But the reality is that you are unlikely to be doing as much as you did before cancer – at least not straight away. You may have to fight yourself to take off your 'filter glasses' and actually recognise the things you are managing to do each day.

EXERCISE

Keep an activity record

Write down everything that you did today. This will help you to understand how much you actually achieve when you think you've done nothing. Here's how:

1. **Break your day up into blocks** – morning, afternoon, evening, night. In each block, jot down two or three things that you did in this stretch of time. This can include 'got out of bed', 'brushed teeth', 'spoke to Mum', 'checked email', 'read magazine', 'made cup of tea'.

2. **Grade how much effort each task involved.** Give each task a number from 0 to 10, where 0 is no effort and 10 is huge effort. Think carefully: on a good day before cancer, making a cup of tea might have scored 0 or 1. But when you're feeling unwell or depressed, making a cup of tea might involve effort levels of 7, 8 or beyond. This will give you a context – the task may seem trivial, but you actually achieved something because it took a lot of effort.

3. **Record how much you enjoyed the task**. Use the same scale (0 to 10, where 0 is not at all and 10 is you loved doing it).

4. **Do this every day for two weeks** – or more – if you can manage it.

Why bother?

Keeping an activity record will help you to realise that you actually do more than you think you do. Over time, you will notice your enjoyment scores may start to go up a bit, and your effort scores start to go down. This change in scores – even if it's small – is very important when you're thinking 'I hate my situation; I don't enjoy anything any more'. Sometimes you need to see evidence to know that things are getting better.

TIP ▶

GET A NOTEBOOK

Using a notebook (or electronic device) rather than scraps of paper will give you a handy record and help you to monitor your progress, because you can look back and see how you've changed.

Step 5: Set fun goals

A vital part of kicking depression is to do things you actually enjoy. You need treats, fun stuff: activities that make you feel good. This is not an optional extra, and it's not selfish. It is completely central to overcoming low mood and depression.

But it can be surprisingly hard to set goals when you're feeling low. It might feel difficult to come up with anything you'd enjoy at all. It can be a good idea get someone close to you to help you to set some goals for yourself – identify things you want to start doing again, things that right now you think you can't face.

EXERCISE

What do I like doing?

Take a look back at your activity record. It's likely to be much fuller than you thought it would be. But what is it full of? Work? Housework? Looking after other people? When you feel low the last things you think about (let alone do) are fun things you might enjoy or that give your life meaning. But these are the key to beating depression. So, even if you looked at this section title and thought either 'There is nothing I like doing' or 'I don't deserve to do what I like doing', don't skip this. Try to read on.

You need to start doing things that you enjoy as well as all those day-to-day tasks. By setting yourself some 'fun goals' you can help yourself to start enjoying life again.

How to set your fun goals

1. **Think about the different areas of your life**, including work, leisure, family, spirituality, fitness, socialising, education or learning and hobbies.

2. **Focus on one fun goal.** Make it an important one – pick either something you used to do, which you liked, but have dropped since cancer, or consider starting something new that you've always wanted to try.

3. **Can you achieve that goal today?** If so, that's great. But many goals take more time. You'll probably need a series of steps or shorter term goals to get there. In Chapter 1: Worries, pages 33–5, Sarah's ultimate goal was to go into the hospital without getting in an anxious sweat. But first she had to establish a set of steps, a 'ladder' of short-term

goals towards her ultimate long-term goal. Setting fun goals works the same way.

4. **Look at your long-term goal and work out the steps you need to get there**. For example, if you want to get back to knitting baby clothes the first steps may be finding your old knitting needles, buying some new wool and ordering a pattern book. The next steps may be practising your basic stitches, starting off with a scarf, before moving on to the ultimate goal of booties and bobble hats.

SMART goal setting

The most important thing is that your goals should be realistic. You don't want to set yourself up for failure. A good trick is to look at what you've chosen as a goal, and to make sure that it is **SMART**:

- **Specific**: Be clear about it – don't just say 'go out more', but 'spend a day at the beach'.

- **Measurable**: How will you know if you've achieved what you set out to do? (Did I spend X minutes or hours on the beach?)

- **Achievable**: Spending a whole day out of the house may be your ultimate goal, but start small – half an hour on the beach may be much more achievable at first. Don't set yourself up for failure.

- **Relevant**: Only pick goals that are meaningful to you (the beach is a place I love – I've had tons of happy times there and the kids love it).

- **Timely**: Ask yourself 'Is now really the right time to work on this goal?' (If it's November, then a day on the beach might be awful – maybe you could postpone that one until summer.)

TIP ▶

KEEP AT IT

You're probably not going to enjoy aiming for your goals at first. It may not feel like 'fun' at all. But if you keep going with your activity record – keep a record of the effort it took to achieve each step, and how much enjoyment you got – then you'll realise that you are making progress. Gradually, you'll start to enjoy the process, and look forward to it – though this can take time.

CASE STUDY

Keith, 45, leukaemia survivor

Goal setting

Keith's plans for setting up a residential home after his leukaemia treatment finished took a massive knock. His bank manager told him and his wife Sylvia that he would not fund their business plan. Keith felt very low. He no longer wanted to work on his beloved motorbike, see his friends or go back to his local darts team, which had previously been a source of great pleasure to him. He became withdrawn and irritable. And he felt guilty, thinking, 'I should be able to snap out of this, I'm no fun to be around, this is so ungrateful to the doctors, nurses and Sylvia who looked after me so well.' He kept going to work, but couldn't see that this was an achievement, and constantly said unhelpful and harsh things to himself ('I should be doing more', 'Anyone can just go to work').

Keith kept an activity record for me, which showed him that he'd stopped doing virtually everything that he used to enjoy. He wasn't convinced that he'd ever enjoy anything again, but he reluctantly agreed to try and get his social life going again. ➜

He decided that he would go to his local pub on Friday night for half an hour. This took enormous effort (he scored his effort a 10) because he wanted to stay at home, not talk to anyone and watch TV. He went anyway. His friends were delighted to see him but he felt awkward and shy and thought he had nothing to say. He did manage a game of darts but he left after twenty-five minutes and was relieved to get out. Even though this was his first trip to the pub in over a year, he saw it as a failure because he had left five minutes before his planned time and he hadn't enjoyed it.

When we met the following week we talked about the score he gave for effort (10). This was evidence that in fact Keith's evening wasn't a failure at all. He'd achieved something massive, just by being there. Keith could also see his thought traps, 'all or nothing thinking'. He didn't stay as long as planned so he'd 'failed'. It had gone 'wrong' so there was no point in trying again. His 'filter glasses' also made him focus on what went wrong (he did not enjoy it), rather than the achievement of having got up and gone in the first place.

Having initially said to me that he'd never set foot in the pub again, Keith reluctantly agreed to try again the following week. But this time Keith thought about how to make his goal more SMART. He aimed for twenty minutes in the pub. He realised it would be more relevant if Sylvia came with him. He also worked out that it was better to go on a Thursday when the pub wasn't so busy.

Over time Keith found that his effort levels dropped and his pleasure levels rose. He managed to increase the time he spent there, go on a Friday night, join in with the darts and feel involved with his friends again. He started to love his weekly pub night again, and his mood improved enormously.

Depressed thinking

How to identify your depressed thoughts

In Chapter 1: Worries, you learned how to be a thoughts and behaviour detective.

When you are feeling depressed, these skills come in very handy. If you identify unrealistic or unhelpful thoughts you can question and change them.

Here's how to identify your depressed thoughts:

1. Look back over your day to pinpoint a time when you felt particularly low.

2. See if you can identify the words that went through your mind at this point.

3. Write them down. This may be difficult or painful if you don't like writing or if your thoughts were upsetting. But by writing the thoughts down you don't just become more aware of them – you become a bit distanced from them too. Note down how you felt and what you did when you had that thought. Again, this will help you to become more aware of the power of your thoughts. You'll notice how they influence your feelings and behaviour.

4. Remind yourself, again, that thoughts are usually just your perception or interpretation of events and not facts (see page 17).

TIP ▶

WRITE IT DOWN

You aren't going to get rid of bad thoughts simply by writing them down, but if they're on paper, somehow your mind will feel that it doesn't have to keep repeating them so much. This really does work.

How to challenge your depressed thoughts

Having spotted and written down your unhelpful or unrealistic thoughts you can now see what thought traps you're falling into (see pages 18–19 for a list of the common thought traps with depression). Gradually, you will learn to spot the traps the moment you fall into them – you won't have to write them down, you'll automatically start to question them.

Once you've spotted your depression thought traps, try asking yourself questions about them.

- **Am I wearing 'filter glasses'** that stop me from seeing things I'm actually achieving, pleasure I have felt and so on?

- **Do I blame myself** for everything that goes wrong but think anything that goes right is a fluke or down to the kindness/support of others?

- **What would I say to someone else** in this situation? (It's amazing how many of us have double standards: one harsh rule for me and one realistic rule for everybody else.)

- **Am I calling myself names** or giving myself labels? Is this fair and does this help me to get going again or feel better?

- **Am I using lots of phrases**, such as 'I should, must, ought to' and so on? These are clues that you are setting yourself lots of expectations. Would you ask someone else to do what you are asking yourself to do? Are you taking your context into account? This isn't about making excuses or lowering your standards. It's about recognising what you've been through.

EXERCISE

Courtroom drama

You've been your own thought detective; you've identified the traps and interrogated them. Now it's time to put those depressed thoughts on trial.

- Write one unhelpful thought down.
- Draw a line dividing your paper in half.
- On one side of the line write down all the evidence to support that unhelpful thought.
- On the other side of the line write down all the evidence against that thought.
- Now it's up to you to come to a judgement: which thoughts are really accurate, fair and helpful? Which thoughts will help you to pick yourself up, set a goal, achieve that goal and beat your way out of the jungle of depression?

CASE STUDY

Sophie, 19, bone cancer survivor

Overcoming depression

Sophie was 17 and in her first year at college studying French and German when she was diagnosed with bone cancer. She took a year out while being treated. She was referred to me a year after her treatment had ended because she had not returned to her course. She was depressed.

→

The first thing we did was set up some 'grieving time' (see page 60). Sophie needed to talk about all the losses her cancer had caused – the disruption, the pain, the damaged relationships, her sense of being left behind by her peers, her backwards step when she moved back home to her parents, her concerns about her appearance and her fertility, her fears for the future, her feelings of uncertainty and her sorrow. She realised that acknowledging her sad feelings wasn't the same as being 'weak, spoilt or selfish'.

Sophie was also well and truly glued to her filter glasses. She said she did 'next to nothing' with her days and that what she did do was 'pretty pointless'. Her activity record was an eye opener: although Sophie was not back at college or socialising much (the things she felt she 'should' be doing), she was really quite busy. She was living with her parents and helped her mother each day with her small greetings card business, which she ran from home. She visited her blind grandfather every other day for tea and to read the newspaper to him. She swam in her local pool three times a week and was reading novels and playing computer games.

Some of her tasks, such as helping her mother, took a considerable amount of effort (scores of 7 to 9) and only gave low levels of enjoyment (1 to 3). But others, including visiting her grandfather and reading, took less effort (4 to 6) and gave her more pleasure than she had realised (scores between 5 and 7). Her activity record also showed her the thought traps she'd fallen into. She realised she had very high expectations: 'I should be back at university'; 'I should be having a great time'. Her filter glasses made her feel she was achieving nothing ('I am only helping Mum stuff envelopes; a baby could do it'). And she was often having 'all or nothing' thoughts: 'All my friends are at university, my life is pointless'.

→

Sophie worked hard at questioning her thoughts. She gradually learned to spot and challenge her thought traps. She then used goal setting to work out that she didn't actually want to go back to college. She realised that what she really wanted was to be a hair and beauty therapist. She set these goals:

- **Long-term goal**: train as a beauty therapist.

- **Medium-term goal**: find out information about local courses and apply.

- **Short-term goal**: get some voluntary part-time work in the local hair and nail salon.

When I last saw Sophie her expectations for herself were reasonable, she could give herself credit for her achievements and knew how to set realistic (SMART) goals (see page 70). She had enrolled on a hair and beauty course and made some new friends. 'I feel so much better,' she told me. 'I'm doing what I want to do rather than what other people want me to do or what I think I should be doing.' Six months later Sophie called to say that she had a job with a hairdresser who was a breast cancer survivor herself. They were setting up a hair and beauty business specialising in services for people with or after cancer.

TIP ▶

DON'T BEAT YOURSELF UP

Writing things down can be tough for many people. When you're feeling low or depressed you may be telling yourself that you are no good at writing. Dredging up the motivation to pick up a pen may be too hard. You might be wondering 'What's the point?' Well, when you write things out, the thoughts are no longer shapeless words rushing through your mind. They are visible in front of you in black and white. If you can see something, you can challenge it.

But if writing is just not for you at the moment don't beat yourself up. There are plenty of suggestions in this chapter that don't require any writing at all – and they are also good ways to improve your mood ('time to grieve', 'eat well', 'exercise', 'goal setting', 'soothe yourself'). When it comes to thoughts, if you don't want to write anything down, just read the section above and have a go in your head.

Anti-depressant medication

When you're caught in the vicious circle of depression it can be very hard to pull yourself out. For some people, especially those who are very depressed, medication ('antidepressants') can kick-start a recovery process, and this can be very helpful. Others are keen to avoid taking any additional medication, perhaps because they want to avoid any side effects of anti-depressants. The strategies outlined in this chapter are usually enough to overcome most low mood and depression. But some people will certainly benefit from medication.

Modern antidepressants are not addictive. But the risk is that you'll think that any progress you make is due to the tablets rather than your own efforts. Elsa, 67, lung cancer survivor, wanted to stop taking antidepressants. She'd been on them for over two years since starting her cancer treatment, and she didn't feel depressed any more. But she was worried that the depression would come back if she stopped. 'I felt so wretched before I took my tablets,' she says. 'They helped me so much, I didn't want to go back to feeling miserable when I stop.'

Elsa hadn't realised that while the tablets did help her to be more motivated, it was Elsa, not the tablets, who got through treatment, rebuilt her physical strength, got herself back to activities that she enjoyed such as volunteering in a local charity shop, doing tapestry and bird watching. Elsa very sensibly asked for advice about stopping her antidepressants. She was able to cut down gradually, keeping herself active and making sure to recognise her achievements (see page 67). 'I took my last little tablet with barely a worry,' she says. 'I knew it had done its job and that I'd cope and be fine without it.'

And finally ... make a soothing list

Overcoming down feelings can be hard work, and you need to give yourself positive, enjoyable, soothing time too. Ask yourself:

- What helps me to relax?
- What helps me to feel soothed and calm?

Draw up a list of things that make you feel calm and peaceful. Doing the list in your head is fine but if you choose to blow it up, laminate it and stick it on the fridge that's a great idea too – the point is to actually do these things for yourself.

It can be simple things like putting a fresh set of sheets on your bed, drinking a hot cup of tea, stroking your cat, listening to music, watching your children or grandchildren play, having a pint in your local (after checking with your medical team, of course). Every day, try to do one thing from your soothing list. Again, this approach is not fluffy or self-indulgent. It is backed up by proper scientific research: studies show that soothing yourself like this will help to tackle your low mood.

Family, friends and carers: How you can help someone who is depressed

If you are trying to support a cancer survivor who is feeling low, then your situation can be almost as difficult and confusing as theirs.

It is normal to feel relieved, happy and excited that their treatment is over. It's also normal to want them to feel good. It can be hell to watch them suffer – again.

It is particularly difficult, this time, when they are feeling low, because there is so little that you can do to help. Sometimes you may feel that everything you try just backfires.

Anila's husband wanted to throw a party for her to give her the chance to see how much her family and friends love her and how proud they are of her (see page 55). But Anila refused to set a date and sometimes even cried if he mentioned it. This was frustrating for him – infuriating sometimes. He just couldn't understand what was wrong with her.

COPING STRATEGY

Ten ways to help a depressed person

1. **Look after yourself** – don't get caught up in a vicious circle of depression too. Make sure **you** are eating, sleeping and exercising. Give yourself treats and pleasures: you're in a very tough situation too and you need to support yourself if you are to look after your loved one.

2. **Examine your own thought patterns** (see page 52). Are you blaming yourself for how the other person is feeling? Are you expecting that you will be able to help them single-handedly? Are you measuring your success purely in terms of the other person's mood? Are you expecting too much from your loved one at this stage?

3. **Focus on what you do achieve** – even if their mood hasn't

changed, remind yourself of all the small and big things you are doing to help them all the time. If you don't do this, it is easy to despair and feel useless.

4. **Get help** straight away if you think there is any danger that they might harm themselves (see pages 58–9). You aren't able to deal with this – it's too much. Your loved one will need expert help at this point. It's worth knowing that the vast majority of cancer survivors **don't** reach this point.

5. **Try not to get into debates or arguments** – you won't 'make' them feel better, and contradicting them is rarely helpful. Anila's husband would frequently tell her she wasn't a failure as a wife and mother but she'd just say 'You don't mean that' or 'You have to say that'. This sort of debate can become demoralising and frustrating for everyone. Try instead to look at the coping strategies listed above and offer to help if they need it – you might be able to help them with goal setting or with their thought traps (though be very careful not to sound like you're accusing them: just offer yourself as someone who can provide an alternative viewpoint).

6. **Try to focus on getting them to be more active**. Low mood and depression can gradually lift when people achieve small, manageable tasks. Instead of supporting the depressed person by doing everything for them, which is natural when you see them struggling, see if you can find tasks for them to do – particularly things that help you. This could range from making you a cup of tea, to helping you decide what to plant in your hanging basket, to looking after grandchildren for an hour. But be very aware that low mood and depression is exhausting – so be careful not to overload your loved one with tasks. It's a fine balance.

7. **Be the 'evidence provider'**. Make realistic, specific comments that are attached to particular things your loved one does or says. When Anila's husband said 'Thank you for

that delicious dinner' or 'I really appreciated you coming with me to visit my parents', he was bolstering her in a clear, labelled way. Anila might not acknowledge it at the time, but his comments gave her 'evidence' to challenge her unhelpful thoughts about herself.

8. **Don't mind read or make assumptions about what the other person wants or needs from you**. It's OK to acknowledge that they seem low and to ask them what support they need, however. When he asked her what she **did** want from him, Anila told her husband that she needed him to help her to gradually contact family and friends. So, he arranged smaller family gatherings outside the family home. They developed a code to use so she could tell him when she needed to leave. A year later they had a party in their home for their daughter's eighteenth birthday.

9. **Remember, you aren't their therapist**. You are too closely involved. But you can try to be a good and non-judgemental listener. Just letting them talk is invaluable – this is how people often come up with their own coping strategies. It might seem you're getting nowhere, and are going over old ground, but keep it up. It's OK, and indeed can be helpful, to give your own opinion about a situation. Don't make it a direct challenge, though: present it as your personal perspective and, at the same time, acknowledge their alternative point of view. Agree to disagree (be nice about it).

10. **Be patient**. Overcoming low mood and depression takes time – how much time varies widely from person to person. Your loved one might not realise they are making progress, and you can help them recognise this. Sometimes it will feel like two steps forward and one step back but do try to notice and hold on to even the smallest signs of progress.

CHAPTER THREE

ANGER

> 6 If one more person says to me that I am so lucky to
> have got through my cancer, I won't be responsible for my
> actions. Yes I've survived and I'm immensely relieved about
> that, but to suggest that I'm lucky to have had my breast
> removed, gone through chemo, lost my hair and had an
> early menopause just shows how ignorant most people are
> about cancer. 9
>
> GILL, 46, BREAST CANCER SURVIVOR

What is anger?

This may well be the sort of question that infuriates you – and
who can blame you? – but it is, in fact, not as odd as it sounds.
In order to effectively deal with your anger, it's a good idea to
understand more about how it works for you.

The anger instinct

Anger is a natural and normal human emotion. It is part of
the body's so-called 'fight–flight mechanism': when facing a
threat your instinctive response is either to fight it, or to run

away. A threat can come in many forms, including that feeling of outrage when something unfair happens, or some unspoken rule is broken.

Basically, anger is the instinct that gets you pumped up enough to tackle (or escape from) the threat. These days, most threats don't actually need a physical response at all. But when we get angry our bodies still get ready for action: it's a pure, animal instinct.

Why does cancer make you angry?

The simple answer is that cancer feels like one hell of a threat to your survival, no matter what your doctor says. Anger is also a natural response to loss – and cancer brings many losses. So, it's little wonder that most people feel some kind of rage or fury during diagnosis and treatment.

'I've led a good and healthy life, tried to do everything right, always put others before myself and the cancer has hit me,' says Terry, 61, liver cancer survivor. 'But my neighbour down the road is the biggest waste of space I know. He drinks, smokes, takes drugs, disrupts this neighbourhood with his shouting, swearing and music blaring out, beats his wife up – and there he is, no health problems at all, living the life of Riley. I can't stop thinking, why didn't he get cancer instead of me?'

Think back to the time of your treatment. There are probably a lot of situations that annoyed you: a thoughtless remark from a colleague, all that waiting around during hospital visits, another bill dropping through your letterbox. Your own thoughts and questions, many of which are unanswerable ('Why me?', 'It's not fair', 'What have I done to deserve this?'), probably made you feel angry and helpless at times too.

But during treatment, anger can be a surprisingly useful emotion. It is very common for people to develop what psychologists call 'a fighting spirit'. They approach the disease

with great determination: they get hold of as much information as they can, work brilliantly with their medical team,
follow instructions to the letter, carry out their own research,
adapt their lifestyle to boost their chances of recovery. They
really give it everything they've got.

During particularly tough moments, the anger – that feeling of being revved up and ready for action – can even help
some people to cope better. 'I did get furious during treatment,' says Maisie, 59, lymphoma survivor. 'It all felt so
unfair, watching my friends and family carrying on with their
lives while mine was put on hold. Whenever I felt this way,
though, I tried to channel it inwards, as if I was sending angry
beams into my body to zap the cancer cells along with the
chemotherapy.'

Anger during cancer treatment, in other words, is normal
and sometimes useful. But afterwards it's a whole different
ball game.

Anger after cancer

But why am I still angry?

You've faced your cancer and you're where you've longed to be.
So why are you still angry? Why, in fact, might you feel even
angrier now than you did during diagnosis and treatment?

You are not out of control. Or mad. You are perfectly sane
and normal, because there are loads of reasons why anger
sticks around – or even gets worse – after cancer.

Here are the main reasons.

'I still feel threatened'

Though cancer is no longer an immediate threat, it might still
feel close by. You probably have thoughts and fears about
the cancer coming back: you're only human (see Chapter 1:

Worries, page 39). You may be struggling with the physical and emotional after-effects of the disease and its treatment. And you're probably also dealing with lots of reminders of what you've been through – and all the things you've lost. All this can bring on bouts of fury. 'I feel so totally furious with myself when I am too tired to do what I used to do before cancer hit,' says Gwen, 77, bladder cancer survivor. 'It's like I can't escape what it's done to me, even now, when it's supposedly over.'

'I feel helpless'

During treatment, you and your medical team are busy doing something about the cancer. But when you reach the end of your active treatment phase, even though it's obviously what you've been longing for, you can end up feeling a bit lost – maybe even helpless. You aren't tackling something head on any more. And this, in turn, can trigger angry feelings. 'I couldn't believe that after all the side effects I've had to deal with I didn't actually want to stop my treatment,' says Mike, 66, throat cancer survivor. 'In fact, I kept asking the consultant if she couldn't just give me a single dose of chemo or some other tablets every six or twelve months just to keep this cancer at bay. Chemo has been my lifeline; it has kept me alive. The doctors just don't understand what it means to me. I feel so angry with them for not understanding and with myself for not being able to persuade them.'

'Other people drive me mad'

Other people's expectations can be frustrating. Whether they assume you'll instantly spring back into your normal life, or insist on treating you like a fragile flower, it's common to feel misunderstood. 'My friends almost start to whisper when I enter the room, as if I am so vulnerable that I can't be spoken to at full volume. It drives me mad,' says Sharon, 31, melanoma survivor. 'I don't understand why they treat me so differently or how on earth I can get them to see that I am OK.'

'I can't stop looking back'

When active treatment ends, people very often begin to look backwards, trying to work out what caused their cancer. It's common to go over and over this. If you smoked, drank too much alcohol, worked around asbestos, ate red meat, lived near a pylon or, indeed, did any of the numerous carcinogenic things we all do every day, then you might feel regret and guilt. You may also feel angry at yourself. 'I was so stupid as a teenager; I wanted to look cool and thought that smoking would do it for me. Then in my twenties and thirties, even when I knew the risks, I just carried on because I thought I was invincible,' says Otis, 52, mouth cancer survivor. 'Cancer happens to other people, not me. Well, what a fool I was, because then it happened to me.'

Similarly, if you – or any healthcare professionals – missed the signs of cancer before your diagnosis then you may feel bouts of fury and regret. 'I was so embarrassed about the smelly discharge that stupidly I left it for ages just hoping it would go away,' says Shonelle, 27, cervical cancer survivor. 'Then when I did go to the GP she just kept asking about my sexual life, and referred me to a sexually transmitted diseases clinic even though I told her I'd only ever had two sexual partners. If she'd examined me properly instead of treating me like that, maybe they'd have caught the cancer sooner.'

'I get frustrated with myself'

Your expectations – 'to get back to normal', 'put the cancer behind me', 'be strong', 'get on with life' – can give you something to aim for. But if you get too fixated on your expectations, they can also become a real pressure. When you're struggling to reach them you get angry with yourself. 'The cancer has disrupted enough of my life and I'm determined not to let it upset me now it's gone,' says Dennis, 63, thyroid cancer survivor. 'But I get so frustrated when I have a down day; it feels like I'm letting it back into my life and I hate being so weak.'

'I'm just angry with the cancer!'

You may just feel angry with the cancer itself. You might be furious about the fear, pain and chaos it brought into your life; livid because it knocked you off course; bitter about all the things you've lost. Maybe you feel like you've been viciously attacked, but there is no attacker to hit back at; no justice system to pursue, nowhere to channel your fury. 'I just hate this disease, I loathe it, despise it, wish I could wipe it off the face of the earth. But what can I do about it?' says Sally, 60, breast cancer survivor. 'Set up a coffee morning fund raising for Cancer Research? That seems so little. I feel so helpless and the anger just eats me up inside, I can almost feel it working its way through me.'

When is anger a problem?

Anger is not always a bad thing. There are certain situations where it's quite useful to get angry: it can help you to respond quickly to a threat, or motivate you to challenge something unfair, or make sure that your needs are met. It's perfectly reasonable, for instance, to be angry if you hear that the local chemotherapy suite is closing. You might use your anger to write letters to the authorities, lobby the people in power, set up a campaign to keep it open.

Anger only really becomes a problem when:

- it becomes a habit
- you see threats or injustices that aren't there
- it's out of proportion to the situation you are facing
- it's too explosive or threatening – when you shout or even hit out, putting other people (and maybe yourself) in danger
- it lasts too long – leaves you feeling helpless, out of control
- it's directed at the wrong target – for instance, you hold it in at work but then get furious with people at home.

Uncontrolled, over-the-top or misplaced anger is difficult not just for you, but for the people around you, too. It can be scary and destructive for everyone.

The 'cover up' emotion

Anger does not always come out in the most obvious way – loud, shouty, vicious, aggressive or physically violent behaviour. It can be sneakier. It might show up in your attitude – you may become less tolerant and more irritable. Or it might be the 'slow burn' thing – whatever made you angry in the first place might be long gone, but you suddenly blow up out of the blue at something apparently small and trivial.

If you could open anger up and take a look inside, you'd probably find a lot of other painful emotions lurking in there too: sadness, regret, grief, loneliness, fear, guilt. This is why anger is 'the cover up emotion'. It hides, and distracts you from all these other important and difficult feelings.

How to manage your anger

Understand it: The anger firework

Fireworks don't just explode:

- First, a spark or flame has to light the touch paper.
- Then the fuse (whether it is a long or short one) has to burn up to the body of the firework.
- This lights the packed explosives; the rocket shoots up into the air and – bam! – explodes.

Anger works this way too.

You may not always know it, but each angry incident will have been triggered by something (the spark or flame). This trigger sets off the thoughts or commentary in your head (the fuse). Your body then responds; it goes on 'full alert' (the explosives packed into the firework, ready to blow). It isn't until the very end of this sequence of events that you get what you think of as the 'anger': the explosion – the shouting, door slamming, arguing, throwing things.

CASE STUDY

Liam, 26, soft tissue sarcoma survivor

'I used to be known as the gentle giant,' Liam told me at our first meeting. 'I was physically really strong but I wouldn't hurt a fly. But since my cancer I feel like Jekyll and Hyde. There is still the old me buried deep down, but on top I am just this angry monster. My mum only has to look at me and I'm shouting at her to leave me alone. My girlfriend says I've changed and I've got to get a grip of myself or she might not be able to stay with me. I want to

→

change but I don't know how. This rage just takes over and I don't know what I am saying or why I am shouting. I do know though that I would still never hit anyone.'

Anger like this can be confusing. You might feel scared and trapped. So the first thing that I did with Liam – as I do with all my clients who are struggling with anger – was to help him understand his anger better.

This involves:

- *recognising that anger does not simply come out of the blue*

- *understanding that anger is made up of your thoughts, your body and your behaviour*

- *tackling and improving your control over each one of these.*

It sounds like a complicated business, but really this is the only way to manage your anger properly. So to start with I asked Liam to think about his own 'anger firework' and try to work out how it happens for him.

Liam's triggers (the spark)

Liam realised that there were two main triggers for his anger:

1. *His friends going out socialising when he felt too tired to join them.*

2. *Coming in from work at the end of the day.*

Liam's thoughts (the fuse)

When getting angry, his thoughts would race to the following issues:

- *The unfairness of cancer, how it had held him back at the prime of his life: 'Why me? Why now? I am just getting started*

➡

out in life and it has stopped everything. I should be out there having a great time like everyone else around me.'

- *How it stopped him from getting his own flat (which made coming back to his parents' home a trigger for anger): 'It is like I am a teenager again, living with my parents, having to depend on them again, it is so degrading.'*

Liam's body (the dynamite)

Liam realised he'd control his anger in front of his friends when they were planning their evening out, but his body (like the body of the firework) became very tense when he was doing this, as if packed with explosives. He'd clench his fists, hunch his shoulders and get very hot.

Liam's angry behaviour (the explosion)

As soon as Liam walked through his parents' front door he lost his inhibitions and exploded (verbally) at his mother and girlfriend, calling them names, arguing with them, shouting, almost regardless of what they said or did.

It really upset him to see so clearly that he was taking out his anger on his mother and girlfriend. But he found this exercise helpful because it allowed him to make sense of the anger. It made his anger seem less strange, and more manageable. Liam didn't lose all the anger or his triggers entirely, but he certainly learned to manage his fury far better, using the techniques explained below.

How to manage your triggers

If you can defuse the anger before it really gets started – and even do something about the causes (triggers) of your anger in the first place – then you are well on the way to controlling it.

EXERCISE 1

Identify your triggers

After each angry incident, once you've calmed down, try to look back. Ask yourself: what happened, at the very start, to trigger the anger? What lit the fuse (my thoughts) that led to the explosion (my angry outburst)?

Lots of things can trigger anger: places, people, words, pictures, certain times of the week or day, demands, becoming overloaded with tasks, situations that make you feel guilty, ashamed, scared. You'd be surprised how many ways there are to trigger anger.

TIP ▶

You might find it helpful to keep a list of your particular triggers. You may then start to identify patterns or themes to what 'sets you off'.

EXERCISE 2

Stop the triggers

How to do this:

- **Become aware of them.** Just knowing what the triggers are can give you a sense of distance from them, and this takes away some of their power. Liam, for instance, became particularly observant on a Friday: he'd listen to his colleagues making weekend plans and notice how he was responding. This gave him a sense of distance from the anger.

- **Avoid them**. OK, so throughout this book you are constantly being told not to avoid difficult things. But with anger it works a bit differently. Rather than feeling that you must express your anger all the time – or it will never leave you – it can sometimes help just to remove yourself from, or avoid, the things that make you angry. Liam, for instance, found that if he arranged a lunchtime meeting on a Friday, and didn't have lunch with his friends and colleagues, then he didn't hear them making their weekend plans and so he didn't become so angry.

- **Change them**. It might be possible for you to change either the trigger or the issues that cause the trigger to be there, once you know what it is. For instance, when he realised how furious he was that he was still living with his parents, Liam started flat hunting again, as he had been just before his diagnosis.

COPING STRATEGY

Manage your thoughts

Your thoughts are the fuse. They either whizz up to that explosive-packed firework, or gradually work their way there on slow burn. But one way or another, they get there and you blow. You could call these 'hot' thoughts.

If you can put out your burning fuse/thoughts before they get to the explosives, then you've controlled your anger. These thoughts are often made up of 'thought traps' (see pages 17–19 for a full explanation of how thought traps work).

Six common anger thought traps

1. **Mind reading:** 'They're all so selfish, not one of my friends is thinking about me and the fact that I'm too tired to go out tonight. They've just forgotten that I was ever ill.'

2. **All or nothing thinking:** 'They are going to have a fantastic night tonight and mine is going to be rubbish' or 'There is no point in going out if I don't have as much energy as the lads.'

3. **Taking things personally:** 'My parents like having me at home; they're trying to keep me with them just so they can keep looking after someone.'

4. **Unhelpful or unrealistic expectations (of yourself or others):** 'My girlfriend should know how I feel and not ask me questions when she can see I don't want to talk.'

5. **Labelling (and using over-emotional language):** 'I'm a selfish, ungrateful, out of control monster' or 'The lads are a bunch of thoughtless, heartless, cruel b******s.'

6. **Thinking the worst:** 'I'm such a misery that my girl-friend will leave me. No one will ever want to be with me. I'll end up alone and friendless.'

EXERCISE 1

Spot your hot thoughts

To start with, carry out this exercise a little while after the angry incident, when you have 'cooled down'.

If you had an angry outburst during the day, wait until you're calmer, perhaps later that evening or even the following day, before going back to try and spot what thought set you off. A bit of distance will make sure you're not so hot any more – you don't want it to wind you up all over again. If you had several anger outbursts in the day, pick just one to work through in the evening.

1. **Imagine yourself on film**. See if you can 'replay' the events surrounding your anger in 'slow motion' in your mind's eye. Try to focus particularly on what you were thinking at the time: What thought was 'hot'? What actual words went through your mind? What thought got you wound up? You may find that some of the thoughts you remember actually make you feel tense again – that's a real clue that these are 'hot' thoughts.

2. **Write those hot thoughts down** (while you are doing your slow motion replay). This makes them very clear – you can see in front of you exactly what you are saying to yourself, so it's easier to challenge the thoughts. It will also give you a sense of distance and this can be particularly helpful with anger (it keeps you 'cool' and able to think more clearly about things). But if you hate writing so much that the process of putting pen to paper triggers your anger, then just do this exercise in your mind.

Once you have carried out several 'slow motion replays' at a distance (some hours after the incident has occurred), try spotting the hot thoughts just after an angry incident – or even while one is happening. Obviously, you can't write them down at that moment; it's just a question of becoming aware of the hot thought so you can move on to putting that hot thought out.

EXERCISE 2

Hose down the hot thoughts

So you have caught the 'hot' thought and it's burning a hole in your mind. You now need your fire extinguisher. The only fire extinguisher available (other than literally going to the bathroom and splashing some cool water on your face, which can help) is to use other – better – thoughts.

Try to ask yourself the following questions whenever you notice a hot thought:

- Is this really true?
- Am I making this too personal?
- Is this thought helpful?
- What can I do or say to myself that is more helpful?

Again, writing this down may be useful at the start, but you need to get good at doing this in your mind, because hot thoughts don't tend to wait for a pen and paper. At first, you could try to take yourself to a quiet space for a minute or two, or go for a quick walk, count to ten slowly, or just have a 'bathroom break' when you feel the hot thoughts taking hold.

EXERCISE 3

Cue cards

Get some index cards or small pieces of paper. Jot down some of the more helpful and realistic beliefs that you have established in the hose down exercise above. You could also write down phrases that will help you to keep calm (see list below). If you're a techno type, put them in your Blackberry or iPhone or whatever device you carry with you, so that you can call them up whenever you need them.

Carry your 'cue cards' around with you all the time.

When you notice you are about to face a trigger or that your hot thoughts are burning, look at your cue cards/electronic cues. Just a glance can remind you that there's a different way of thinking.

Examples of cues that people have found useful:

- Most people are not out to get me.

- Things don't have to be perfect.
- Count to ten.
- Slow your breathing.
- I can manage this.

The more often you can look at your cues, the more deeply embedded they become in your mind. Some people say that they get so they just have to touch their cue cards in their pocket, and they feel calmer. Your cues encourage cooler thoughts to kick in when you are facing a trigger. **These cool thoughts are your fire extinguisher.** They hose down the hot thoughts – dampen the fuse – and so the firework rarely blows.

COPING STRATEGY

Manage your body tension

Anger makes your body tense. Relaxing your body is therefore a major part of successfully controlling anger.

The main ways to do this are through exercise and relaxation. Chapter 8: Relax will give you a more detailed set of body calming exercises. But when it comes to anger, a few specific techniques can be particularly helpful:

- **A short and sharp burst of activity**: Your firework (body) is dynamite-packed, primed to blow. But exercise can release that tension – get rid of the dynamite – before the burning fuse reaches it. When you feel you're about to blow, the short, sharp approach works best. Do something that will use up your energy quite quickly. Again, what works for you will very much depend on your physical capabilities, and where you happen to be at the time. People find the following sorts of things helpful: punching a cushion; a brief, brisk walk; digging the garden; star jumps, running up a flight of stairs. If you need to, and can manage to go further, things like taking a run, kicking a football against a wall, doing a set of push ups are useful. You are aiming for something that gets you a little out of breath, just for a short time.

- **Regular exercise**: For longer-term anger control, regular exercise works wonders. It helps you to release underlying body tension. If you are more relaxed generally, your fuse won't be lit so easily, and your explosives won't be as tightly packed – you'll be less likely to get angry. Aim for moderate exercise, ideally three or four times a week (see Chapter 2: Depression and Low Mood, pages 64–6 for ideas). The key is to do the exercise regularly – and, if at all possible, to do something that gives you pleasure and a sense of achievement. If you are physically up to it, you might find sports such as tennis, squash, cricket, football or netball, where you have an opponent, or team, give you a way to channel pent-up angry feelings.

- **Relaxation**: You can learn specific relaxation techniques to use on the spot, when you feel your fury building. You can also practise regular relaxation techniques that – like regular exercise – reduce your underlying tension, making you less likely to get angry in the first place. Chapter 8: Relax explains relaxation techniques in full, but here are the ones that are best for anger.

Try this: Two instant anger-defusing tricks

When the fuse of your anger firework is actually lit and it is burning fast towards the dynamite, here are two tricks to try:

1. **Slow breathing** is a quick way to calm your body and mind and can be done anywhere, any time. The key is to **make**

your out breath longer than your in breath. You can count as you breathe, imagine you are breathing out through a straw, whistle or pretend to blow up a balloon (i.e. purse your lips). With each out breath let your shoulders drop and notice the relaxation flowing through your body.

2. **Squeeze–release** is a simpler version of the muscle relaxation techniques in Chapter 8: Relax. It helps when you're about to explode: simply clench, then release your fists, or hunch up and then release your shoulders. This quickly releases tension. It also gives your hands and arms a useful alternative to lashing out.

Longer-term relaxation methods for anger management

It can help to build calming exercises into your daily routine. Set aside ten to fifteen minutes each day when you won't be disturbed. Lie down and breathe slowly for a minute or two. Then do squeeze–release along with some visualisation (in Chapter 8: Relax). Make sure you choose a setting for your visualisation where you feel cool, calm and collected. Practising this regularly will reduce your overall level of tension and lower the chance that you'll get riled up by an anger trigger.

When you blow anyway

Damage limitation

There are times when no amount of deep breathing is enough. You've tried to control your triggers, to manage and balance your thoughts, to reduce your physical tension but you're going to explode anyway. When this happens, you need damage limitation.

In the short term, you need to contain the explosion – make it less upsetting.

Here are some strategies that many cancer survivors have found useful:

- Walk out of the room: sometimes just physically removing yourself from the thing, situation or person that's making you angry can help.

- Punch a cushion or pillow.

- Tear or scrunch up a newspaper.

- Throw or kick a ball against an outside wall.

- Splash cold water on your face – this can help you 'cool down' quicker.

- Go outside to shout – sometimes you need to voice it anyway.

- Slam a door.

- Say 'I am angry. I need some space. I cannot speak/do what you ask/answer you/make sense right now'.

In the longer term damage limitation means finding ways to communicate your needs and assert yourself in a reasonable way. Assertive behaviour includes being honest and open about your own feelings, but sensitive to the effect your honesty has on the person you are speaking to. It's important to respect yourself here (don't start labelling yourself as a 'bad' or 'weak' person). But you also have to respect other people and their opinions.

Expressing your anger

You may find that if you tend to store your anger up it's hard to get it to just flow away. It goes on and on; the same things bother you over and over. If this sounds like you, try these two techniques to help you 'get it out'.

The empty chair technique

Imagine that the person (or the cancer) you are angry with is sitting in the chair in front of you. Now, take as much time as you need to say all the things that you would really like to say to them, but can't, because you're a civilised grown-up human being (or trying to be). This is your big chance to let rip, shout, swear, use every name under the sun and describe in great detail exactly what you would like to do to them.

> **TIP▶**
>
> It does help to physically get an empty chair to look at – perhaps make sure you are alone in the house for this one – and this can be seriously therapeutic. Repeat this technique as often as you like: you'll know when you've had enough.

The forbidden letter technique

Sit down and write the letter you wouldn't send. Go on – let it all out, be as crazy, hysterical and unreasonable as you like. But never **ever** send it, no matter how much you want to. Destroy it immediately. This is about emotional expression, **not** communication. This technique, and/or the empty chair, might be enough to make you feel you've let the anger out. Or they might be a starting point that helps you to identify things you need to talk about more.

When you need professional help

Understanding and managing anger is a huge challenge for anyone, at any time, let alone after cancer. But anger can be such a destructive emotion, and whether you often keep it to yourself or you express it loudly to people around you, it's important to get it under control.

It's particularly important, however, to control anger if you end up being aggressive or violent. If your anger is leading to dangerous or damaging behaviour either towards yourself or to other people, get help now.

Even if your behaviour doesn't seem too extreme, if you find that you try the anger management strategies in this chapter for a month, and you're still having regular outbursts of anger that leave you or those around you distressed, then getting some professional help can be a really good idea. Talk to your GP or your healthcare team so that they can find you the help you need.

CASE STUDY

Liam, 26, soft tissue sarcoma survivor

The forbidden letter

Liam's girlfriend found an old Buddhist saying: 'Anger is like a hot coal; if you hold it too long you get burnt.'

This struck a chord for Liam. He realised that his anger was hurting not just people around him but also himself. So he came to me for help. He thought the empty chair technique was too weird, but he did use the forbidden letter, and he said it released loads of pent-up anger and frustration. He wrote several letters, to all sorts of people (and to his cancer) and said that one of the best moments was tearing each one up into tiny pieces.

Liam began swimming regularly at a local pool. Then he discovered karate, a martial art that teaches techniques of self-control and self-defence. He became really good at this, even though he had one leg shorter than the other after surgery.

→

The last time Liam and I met he said: 'I still get niggled by day-to-day things that go wrong – things like the photocopier breaking down, or getting stuck in traffic. But I know this is normal and after a bit of slow breathing or muscle squeeze–release, it just fades away. The anger that dominated my first months after treatment has gone now. I think this is because I've found a physical way to get it out – I've cooled my thoughts down, and my fuse isn't short any more.'

Liam told me that he's accepting the fact that cancer happened to him – that there's no rhyme or reason for it. He can control himself better both physically and emotionally, and feels optimistic about the future.

Getting started

All this can sound like a palaver – like yet another thing to have to face, or get done; yet another thing to beat yourself up about. When you're wound up, dealing with so much negativity, feeling short-fused and irritable, the last thing you feel like doing is calmly tackling your anger, stage by stage. But if you can try some of the techniques in this chapter, maybe just pick one or two at first – you will find that they work.

Anger can be draining, embarrassing, distracting – and it can be scary (both for you, and for other people). When you put it behind you – or find ways to cope much better when it happens – then you really can take a huge step forward in your recovery. You'll find that all sorts of areas of your life feel better, from your energy levels, to your relationships. It really is worth having a go. Other people will probably thank you for it, but most of all, you'll thank yourself.

Family, friends and carers: How you can help with anger

1. **Look after yourself**: You may need support too. Watching a loved one feeling angry, or having that anger directed at you, is unsettling, upsetting, worrying and sometimes even scary. It can really help to have someone – ideally a person who is not too involved with your loved one – to talk to about what you are going through. This is not selfish – it's more than OK for you as a carer to need support too.

2. **Try to remind yourself that anger is a natural 'side effect' of cancer**: It might be directed at you but it's unlikely that you're the real 'cause'. It's not easy but try to remind yourself of this as often as you can.

3. **Remind yourself what you appreciate about your friend or family member**: It may even help to write down a list.

4. **Use your own judgement** about when and how to intervene when they are angry – in the immediate moment they may not appreciate your input, but they may welcome it later.

5. **Let them know that you are available to listen** when they are not actively angry. If they do talk to you it is OK to acknowledge and accept their feelings, but not their behaviour. ('I know you feel like life is unfair but when you shout at me, it's very hard for me to handle.')

6. **Set and maintain your own standards**: Work out what you are prepared to accept from their behaviour. It's important to understand why the person is angry but this doesn't mean you have to put up with behaviour that you find unacceptable. It might help to write this down for yourself. By setting, and maintaining, your own standards you will convey a sense of calm, continuity and stability

for your loved one. They may not be able to tell you they appreciate this at the time, but it will be hugely helpful.

7. **Encourage your loved one to get regular exercise and practise daily relaxation techniques** (see Chapter 8: Relax). Offer to exercise with them if you can manage it – take a regular walk or jog, or a relaxation class. This can be incredibly helpful to them, and will also give you a great way to tackle your own tension and emotions.

CHAPTER FOUR

SELF-ESTEEM
AND BODY IMAGE

❝The hair loss was horrendous. I'm a hairdresser, I love hair, but there was my hair, falling out in clumps. I think I found the hair loss worse than anything else in my whole cancer experience.❞

IRIS, 58, UTERINE CANCER SURVIVOR

What is self-esteem and why does it matter?

Your self-esteem is, basically, how you feel about yourself. Of course, this can be quite complicated. We all have various underlying beliefs about ourselves, whether we're consciously aware of them or not. These beliefs influence how we judge ourselves, minute by minute, hour by hour, day by day. They also dictate how we behave: our decisions, actions, judgements; the way we interact with other people, or react to challenges and setbacks. In other words self-esteem is incredibly important – it is a major part of who you are.

If you stop to notice your thoughts for a bit, you'll realise that you're actually making judgements about yourself all the time – in fact, you're probably doing it right now. There's this running commentary going on in your mind about how you are doing, what you think of yourself, your body, how others view you. Sometimes this is helpful. Sometimes it isn't. But it is definitely not set in stone.

In fact, self-esteem is quite fragile: it changes all the time. Your personal history, along with whatever is going on for you right now, keep it in a state of flux. Of course, cancer brings huge challenges, upheavals and changes in your life. It's not surprising, then, that most cancer survivors at some point realise their self-esteem has taken a knock.

This can be hard to come to terms with. It can be genuinely difficult to move on with your life if you feel that a fundamental part of yourself is not the same. The good news is that there are many ways to rebuild your self-esteem. You might even end up stronger than you were before. This chapter is going to show you how.

Body image and why it matters too

Your body image is the picture you have of your physical self. This picture might be loosely based on facts and figures – your health, strength or vital statistics. But it is also heavily influenced by your judgement, and how you interpret things. This means that your body image is closely bound up with your self-esteem.

You take the external 'evidence' – for instance, facts about your body's health or appearance – and you interpret it. Often you'll change these facts completely as you do so. This is going on all the time, whether you're aware of it or not.

Cancer almost always brings bodily changes: sometimes radical ones. You might feel that your relationship with your body has changed dramatically since your diagnosis. Some cancer survivors feel that they barely recognise their own bodies after treatment.

This can affect not just how you see yourself physically, but also how you feel about yourself – and, therefore, how you behave. Your changed body image, in other words, can affect anything from your relationships to your career to your entire sense of who you are.

This chapter will help you to tackle the changes to your self-esteem and your body image. It will help you to adjust, get to know yourself, communicate how you feel about all this to others (who may be far less aware of the changes than you are) and ultimately move on with your life.

Cancer survival and body image

Your bodily changes may be visible to others – or they may be more subtle and private. You might feel that these physical changes are relatively manageable: you are adapting, you are coping. Or, the changes to your body might feel like an assault on your very identity, a kind of bereavement. They might feel unreasonable and not manageable at all.

Perhaps the way you feel about your changed body lies somewhere in between these extremes. Either way, it can help to understand just what has happened, and to have some coping strategies up your sleeve.

Visible physical changes post-cancer may include:

- hair loss, followed by changes in the way your hair grows, its colour or texture

- weight gain or loss

- loss of a limb

- changes to mobility

- changes to, or loss of voice

- scars.

Physical changes that may be hidden, but are just as profound:

- colostomy bags
- swallowing difficulties
- port-a-caths *in situ*
- a missing breast (or two)
- a reconstructed breast (or two)
- other scars beneath clothes.

Loss and vulnerability

Physical changes to your body often go hand in hand with psychological changes – changes to the way you see your body, and also to your self-esteem. Many cancer survivors say they are left with an unfamiliar sense of loss and vulnerability because of the physical changes they've gone through.

If you always thought of yourself as healthy, strong and able, it's easy to feel exposed after cancer. Before diagnosis, many people don't even realise that they feel physically invincible. But actually most healthy people feel, to some extent, like nothing can go really wrong with their body. This belief is a very useful brain tool: it helps us get through life without being crippled by health worries. Age tends to erode this – but with ageing, the change is gradual.

A life-threatening illness such as cancer fast-forwards this process. Wham! One minute you're healthy, the next you're diagnosed and the image you unconsciously carried round of yourself as a healthy person is blown out of the water.

Who am I now?

'All I had was a sore throat, just like countless ones I'd had before. I only went to the GP because my voice didn't come back completely. I thought she was going to say it was tonsillitis. But she sent me to the hospital straight away. It was cancer of my larynx,' says Andy, 52. 'I still can't get my head around how that could happen to me. I'd always been perfectly healthy. I thought you were ill with cancer, but I was fine; it was nothing out of the ordinary.'

Where has the trust gone?

Your body has let you down. It's no longer the reliable, trusty companion it once was. It has become something you don't know or understand. Perhaps even something to fear.

Since body image and self-esteem are bound up together, a change like this will also dent your self-esteem: you aren't the person you once were.

CASE STUDY

Jamal, 35, testicular cancer survivor

Self-esteem

Jamal, a paramedic and new dad, found that his self-image took a big knock when he was diagnosed with testicular cancer. Jamal has always been immensely fit and healthy – a keen runner, rarely ill, always last to bed, and first up in the morning. The treatment went well, but Jamal was left feeling that he no longer knew his own body and certainly could not trust it any more. When I saw him, a year after his treatment finished, he was feeling lost.

'When I was given my diagnosis I kept thinking: I am a man of 35, I have just had my first child, I'm young and strong, just starting out. I can't have cancer, this doesn't happen to people like me,' Jamal told me. 'I couldn't relate this diagnosis to the body I thought I had – the person I thought I was. And I still can't. After

→

surgery, when I was still mostly confined to bed, I found myself thinking that I couldn't be a strong, active dad to my newborn son. I also felt that I could never go back to work as a paramedic because the tables had turned: I wasn't the helper any more; I needed help myself. Now I'm back at work but I know that I'm not contributing the way I did before. I used to be able to motivate my colleagues, make them laugh, but now I just put my head down and get on with the job.'

This loss of confidence is so common, post-cancer. Jamal realised that he had multiple roles – as a spouse, parent, friend, worker, provider, carer, joker, leader, organiser, peace-maker and colleague. These roles, on the surface, had not changed. But the way he felt about his ability do them had changed a lot.

I explained to Jamal that it can take a very long time to adjust. He needed time to get to know this 'new self'. And he needed support, to rebuild his confidence. We worked together, using the methods described in this chapter. Jamal found 'Permission to Grieve' (page 113–14) a particularly useful starting point. The pressure to 'move on' was immense, he said, and everyone kept telling him how 'lucky' he was. But he badly needed time to face, and feel sad for, what he'd lost. He was reluctant at first, saying it seemed 'self-indulgent', but when he allowed himself the chance, he found it a huge release. Jamal also found the 'case for the defence' exercise (pages 130–1) helpful to catch his own 'thought traps' and correct them. He now feels he is far less hard on himself. All this took time and effort, but Jamal did adjust. 'I don't feel like the same person I was before,' he says now. 'I've changed – my attitude to life, my job, my roles – everything. But I do feel I understand these changes far better, and can accept them (and explain them to others). It's ongoing, but nowadays, at least I feel I can do it: I can be a good dad, paramedic and husband. Not the one I was before, but the one I am now.'

Recognising what you've been through

The first step you need to take is to recognise the changes (mental and physical) that you've gone through, from treatment to post-treatment.

During treatment you had a goal; a kind of map to follow. You had your medical team for support, advice and direction. Whatever you were going through, you were in some way focused and supported. But after treatment, you're more alone. There's that unmapped future stretching ahead of you. How do you tackle it?

The end of treatment is a time when the changes to your body image and self-esteem can become hardest to handle – even harder than during treatment.

- It begins to sink in that some of the physical changes you've faced are long term.

- As you get back to your life – your old roles and responsibilities – you can't stop looking back to the way you used to be.

'I used to be able to run my dog grooming business without any administrative help,' says Judy, 49, bladder cancer survivor. 'I was organised and efficient back then. But now I am so changed that I find it's all I can do to groom the dogs. I have had to get a girl in to help with the diary and accounts.'

PERMISSION TO GRIEVE

- Give yourself permission to think about, and feel sad about, what you've lost. This isn't self-indulgent. It's really necessary if you're to feel better about yourself.

- Let yourself think about the things that have changed – look at old photos or films of yourself.

- Express how you feel about this creatively if it helps: use prose, poetry, painting, music or anything that works for you.

- Find someone to talk to about your loss and sadness. Maybe you have a partner or close friend who could listen to you, but if this feels too close to home, you might be able to talk to someone less close to you: the physio you're seeing to rebuild your strength; one of the nurses on your cancer team or at your GP's surgery; the pharmacist you've got to know throughout your treatment; a religious or spiritual guide. Cancer support services are also very used to talking to people whose confidence has taken a bashing. They can offer support either in person or over the phone. If you have access to the internet, you'll also find that cancer support websites and chat rooms are filled with people who are going through similar things. It can really help to talk about what you've lost.

- If talking's just not for you – even anonymous talking – that's fine too: as long as you talk to yourself and let yourself grieve for what's gone.

See page 60 for more on setting aside a time to 'grieve'.

See page 60 for more on setting aside a time to 'grieve'.

TIP ▶

PINK ELEPHANTS AGAIN

Yes, we're back there: trying not to think about something only makes it more likely to crop up again (see pages 29–30). Here's what to do:

- Watch out for thoughts that may be telling you that it's

ungrateful, spoilt, indulgent or dangerous to think about what you have lost, when you could have lost your life.

• Instead, think about what you'd say to a friend or loved one in this situation. Tell yourself, as you (hopefully) would a friend: 'It's OK to think like this. You've been through so much and you have lost a lot – give yourself some time to get through this.'

A common reaction: Avoidance

As human beings, we are brilliant at protecting ourselves from a threat. When faced with something difficult that makes you anxious, your instinct is probably to try to avoid it. You may find you've stopped doing things you used to enjoy, not because you can't manage them physically, but because you've lost confidence. This is one significant reason why many people become more isolated after cancer.

You may be wondering, at this point, how it's possible to 'avoid' either your body or self-image – after all, they're with you all the time aren't they? But people are great at inventing ways to stop themselves from facing the changes they've been through. Maybe you keep your eyes fixed forwards when you walk down the street so you won't catch your own reflection in a shop window. Maybe you get your partner to change your colostomy bag or clean the site, because you can't face looking and need to distract yourself instead.

Avoidance tactics (see Chapter 1: Worries, pages 27–8) can work in the short term. They stop you getting 'set off' by things, and upsetting yourself unduly. It's totally understandable that avoidance should become your main way to 'cope' post-cancer. The trouble is that these tactics don't work in the long term. When you avoid things, they fester – they don't go away.

COPING STRATEGY

Set gradual goals

The first step is to try to notice the patterns of avoidance you've built up. You can then develop a plan for facing things more constructively.

Of course, you can't expect yourself suddenly to begin to face all the things that are upsetting or scaring you. This isn't realistic. So, the key is to develop a gradual plan that will help you to face, and accept, things you've been trying to avoid.

To do this, you'll need to work out what you're aiming for – your 'goal'. You can then build yourself a kind of 'ladder' of small steps that will slowly get you to that goal.

For instance, if you've stopped going out because you're worried about being stared at, you're not going to cope well if you somehow force yourself to go to a really big party and 'face people'. Instead, you could start by making a list of things you could say to any comments people might make (see pages 119–20). You could then go out, with your partner or a friend, to your local café for just fifteen minutes. Slowly, step by step, you can build up your outings until one day – maybe weeks or even months down the line – you'll be able to face a big party again. And maybe even enjoy it.

CASE STUDY

Tricia, 57, breast cancer survivor

Avoidance

Tricia came to see me two years after finishing treatment for breast cancer. She talked to me about the horror she felt at the scars on her breast. She had undergone a left breast lumpectomy followed by chemotherapy, which she felt she'd managed as

→

successfully as she could have. But she felt physically revolted every time she looked at the scars on her breast. So she looked at them as little as possible.

Tricia got dressed and undressed in the dark. She slept in a bra. She removed mirrors from the bathroom. She showered with her eyes shut. She no longer took baths. She didn't rub emollient creams into her scars and, perhaps most upsettingly of all, she hadn't shown them to her husband, Joe.

We worked out that Tricia's ultimate goal was to feel comfortable enough with her breast scars so that she could allow Joe to look at them. This would help them to be more intimate, physically. So we worked together to draw up her 'ladder'. Tricia decided what each step was to be, and she was in control of when to move from one step to the next.

Tricia's ladder

Step 1: Look at scars for one minute when getting dressed in the morning.

Step 2: Look at scars for two minutes when getting dressed in the morning.

Step 3: Look at scars for five minutes when getting dressed in the morning.

Step 4: Touch scars for thirty seconds while looking at them in the morning.

Step 5: Touch scars for two minutes while looking at them in the morning.

Step 6: Rub emollient/moisturising creams into the scars as recommended by nurse.

Step 7: Put mirrors back in the bathroom and bedroom.

→

Step 8: Have a bath at least three times a week and open eyes when in the shower.

Step 9: Take bra off at night and sleep just in nightdress.

Step 10: Repeat steps 1 to 6 but this time with Joe (husband) doing the looking and then touching.

I told Tricia that each step would feel uncomfortable, awkward and even unpleasant but if she could stick with it, and repeat it daily, she'd find that the negative feelings would fade. Gradually, she'd feel little or no awkwardness. This was the moment when she should move on to the next step.

'To start with it really felt quite horrendous,' Tricia told me. 'The thought of looking at my scars was just so awful. But I knew that I was following a plan, that I only had to stick with it for one minute, and that I really wanted to get over this. I was amazed by how quickly things changed. Within four weeks, instead of being revolted by the scars I was bored by them!'

At our final session, Tricia said: 'I've decided not to go to the plastic surgeon. I've come to accept my scars. I'm never going to like them, but I'm not frightened or dominated by them any more. They're a sign of what I've been through, of the random nature of life, but also of the strength of my relationship with Joe.'

COPING STRATEGY

How to improve your body image

Step 1: Let yourself grieve

Grieving can be a really tough process, and everyone has their own way of doing it. But before you can start to like (or at least not be horrified by) your altered body, it's important to actually grieve for the body you've lost.

Step 2: Coping with comments (or silences)

If your physical changes are visible, then you're likely to come up against questions or comments from people you know; perhaps even from strangers. This can be upsetting, annoying and hard to deal with. Equally, when people you do know say nothing about your changed appearance, their silence can be hard to handle too.

It's helpful to have some ready planned phrases to use in response to the questions, comments or silences. Exactly what you say will depend on who you're facing, and how you feel at that moment.

What to say (and who to say it to)

- **How to open the door.** Plan how you'll respond if the person is someone you'd like to be open with. Ask yourself what level of detail you want to go into. You might need a brief and basic reply: 'I've had cancer and I'm coping with these physical changes, but I'm OK. How are you?' Or, if you do want to talk in more depth you could check if they're ready for this: 'Thanks for asking – I've had a really tough time with cancer as you can see. It would be really good to talk some time. Maybe we can fix a time to meet up?'

- **How to close the door.** Plan what to say to someone you'd rather not talk to. There are different types of answers here, depending on who that person is, and how they approach you. If it's someone you like and value you might want to say something to stall them like: 'Sorry, I just don't feel like talking about all this now.' On the other hand, if the question was nosy or →

just plain rude, then take your pick: have a set of put downs or a simple planned silence tucked up your sleeve so you won't think of the perfect response five minutes after they've moved on. Here are some ideas: 'Do you have a habit of making personal comments?'; 'I have lost my hair/limb/voice/looks but you appear to have lost your manners/humanity/kindness'. The temptation to swear and rant at someone rude or insensitive is sometimes overwhelming. But in general, this sort of conflict will do you no good – it will use up valuable energy and get you nowhere. If you can manage to ignore it and move on, perhaps just saying your scathing comment to yourself silently, or giving a withering look, you will probably find that you cope better.

- **How to stall**. Remember that your responses might change: how you happen to feel on that particular day really matters. It might be a day when you just don't want to talk to anyone about anything personal. Remember that however much you care about the person asking you the question you don't have to answer them now. Plan what to say if you want to put off answering, without closing the door entirely. ('It's been difficult, and I don't want to talk about it right now, but maybe some time I will.')

- **Giving others the 'heads up'**. If a situation is coming up, perhaps a return to work or an evening out, you could let people know in advance how you'd like them to respond to your changed appearance. Perhaps you (or your boss?) could send out an email. Or you could text your friends. Many people feel awkward and lost, and they just don't know what to say or do, so they'll really welcome your advice.

TIP ▶

BE KIND TO YOURSELF

It's important not to pressurise yourself to adjust. You can't expect to get used to your changed body overnight. Body image is a slowly evolving process at the best of times and if you've had to face big changes to your body, virtually overnight, then it takes time to adapt. It's unrealistic and unfair to expect yourself to accept things instantly.

CASE STUDY

Judy, 49, bladder cancer survivor

Coping with questions

Judy wasn't coping well with the things people would say – or not say – about her changed appearance (her short hair). Sometimes she'd get angry, sometimes she'd cry, or storm off, or become silent, or gabble with embarrassment, or simply be abrupt. Social interactions were making her feel very stressed and unhappy. Formerly sociable and confident, she began to feel nervy and isolated.

I encouraged Judy to brainstorm a list of possible responses she could give to comments about her short hair. She carried this list round with her in a small notebook, and looked at it regularly so that she'd be prepared.

Her responses included:

- *'It's growing back after chemotherapy.'*
- *'I've suffered some hair loss so I think it looks better short.'*

→

- *'I was having an Annie Lennox moment.'*

- *'I wanted a change.'*

- *'Thanks for noticing.'*

- *'I see you've had a change too (followed by a comment on some aspect of their appearance).'*

- *'Mind your own business.' (Judy wasn't sure she could ever say this to anyone, but it was often her most immediate thought! So, instead she planned to say: 'Actually, it's very personal. I don't want to talk about it, so I'd rather you didn't bring it up again'.)*

For Judy, the silences from her friends were almost more awkward than the random comments from strangers. But she realised that, when she felt like it, she could open up a conversation by turning one of her listed responses into a question.

'I found that if I commented on my own short hair and asked what they thought of it – if I should colour it, or whether I should still be wearing my turban – this opened the flood gates. My friends were so anxious not to say the wrong thing that they ended up not saying anything at all.'

How to rebuild your self-esteem

The changes you've been through can alter your sense of who you are, sometimes radically. Adjusting to this new 'you' can be a complicated process. You're not a patient any more. But you don't feel like your old self either. And how do you do anything about this, when you're physically weakened, or changed?

Coping with other people's expectations

The people around you probably just want you to go back to the way you were before. They might assume that this will happen. But, as you no doubt know all too well, it's just not that simple.

Often, a member of your medical team or a loved one can inadvertently make things worse. 'At my last appointment my consultant shook my hand and said well done, now off you go and get back to being a partner, father and paramedic,' says Jamal, testicular cancer survivor (see pages 111–12). 'Then my own father asked me when I would be winning the Tour de France. I know he ment it as a joke, but I felt as if nobody really understood where I was, or who I was: least of all me …'

It's as if people assume that the minute you walk out of the consultant's office, you'll be back doing what you did before – or doing more, even. Family members and loved ones are looking for something to cling to: they desperately want to feel that you're 'better'; that they have you 'back'.

Of course, you may just bounce back into your old life, or something like it – people do. But most don't. So, if you are struggling, or just trying to work out who, exactly, you're supposed to be, then what you need is time. And a plan.

COPING STRATEGY

Focus on what you are doing

It's all too easy to focus on all the things you're **not** achieving. It's easy to forget that you are recovering from a life-threatening illness. And it's easy to find yourself thinking: 'But I used to be able to do so much more' or 'What's the point of all this?'

When you feel this way, you might be ignoring the things you **are** getting done, day after day. So if you try to focus on what you have done each day (as opposed to all the things you haven't managed) you will realise you're achieving far more than you might think.

EXERCISE

Log your achievements

Try to write down one thing (it can be very small) each day that you've done well, ideally in a notebook. Gradually build up to three or four things every day. This is not about puffing yourself up, becoming big-headed and self-obsessed. It's actually a kind of protection: a way to stop yourself from creating an unfair idea of who you are. It can really help to write this down, perhaps last thing at night, before you go to bed because you'll end up with a record of what you've achieved. This is 'evidence': it forces your brain to recognise that your achievements really do exist. This, in turn, will boost your self-esteem.

You can also create a 'to do list'. Set yourself a goal or set of goals (your 'to do list'). These can be basic ('feed the cat', 'buy a newspaper'). At the end of each day tick off the things you did.

TIP▶

BEWARE THE 'YES BUTS'

We all do this to ourselves – 'Yes, I did go to the shops today but only because there was nothing in the house to eat'. It's as if we just can't let ourselves get too cocky. But there's no danger of that. This is about recognising the small steps you are making every day. If your self-esteem has taken a knock, simple things like writing down your small achievements can work wonders, from the inside out.

EXERCISE

Dig deeper

This exercise shows you a way to understand – and develop – the way you see yourself.

It's worth thinking a bit about the way you see yourself nowadays. This isn't pointless navel gazing. It will help you to understand the deep changes you've been through. This, in turn, will help you to accept these changes, and to get your life back on track.

1. **Ask yourself how you saw yourself** – before cancer. Did you have a strong sense of who you were and of your role in life? How would you describe yourself? ('I'm the provider for my family'; 'I'm the person who organises this family'; 'I'm the joker in the office'; 'I'm a private person who doesn't confide in others'; 'I'm strong and independent'; 'I'm a good-looking person who takes trouble over my appearance'; 'I'm an arty, musical, creative type'; 'I'm a leader'; 'I'm solid and dependable'; 'I'm the person who is busier now I am retired than I was when working').

2. **Now dig deeper.** Is this the full picture? These 'headline' ways of looking at yourself are valuable: they help you to know where you're going; to make sense of who you are and why you do what you do. But they can also dominate your self-image. It's easy to collect all the evidence that backs up this way of looking at yourself, while ignoring the things that point to a different 'you'. Yes, you brought home the biggest pay packet, were a working mother, kept yourself busy in retirement – but what else did you do? Who else are you?

Try asking yourself these questions:

- **What else did I do?** As a family member, friend, colleague what else did I do that wasn't the headline news but was always a part of how I behaved? For instance, were you the person who could defuse a tense situation? Were you good at reassuring others, or making them laugh, in difficult times? Were you practical – could you fix fuses or bake the fancy birthday cake? Did you take your neighbours' dog for a walk or keep an eye on their home while they were away? Were you a shoulder to cry on or a good bloke in a crisis? Would you help a blind person cross a busy street or give a friendly nod to your newsagent as you bought your paper?

- **Is it really all over?** See how this is all in the past tense? Now ask yourself – has it really gone? Certainly some of the headlines might have been wiped out by cancer – maybe you aren't the 'main earner' or the 'multi-tasker' any more – and this can be really horrible. But when you look at yourself more closely there may well be other, subtler parts of yourself that are still going strong. When the chips are down, these lower key, emotional roles in life are more important and more valuable (to you and others) than any of the 'headlines' – the pay packet, the spotless home, the glittering career. At first, your brain will focus on your headline roles when you do this exercise, but if you keep going, you'll realise there's much more to you than that.

TIP ▶

'YES . . . AND'

If you're feeling bad about yourself it's going to be hard to think realistically about who you are, what you do, how you relate to and give meaning to other people. You may well come up with all sorts of unhelpful thoughts about yourself.

That's OK – get through those, let them come out (if you ignore them they're only going to pop back). But then **force** yourself to go further – say to yourself '**yes ... and**': What else do I do? How would a neighbour describe me? What would a friend list as my qualities? Why does a loved one love me? You don't have to tell anyone about any of this – it's just for you. It won't make you big-headed. This is the 'case for the defence' in your own private prosecution – and everyone has the right to a defence (see 'courtroom drama', page 75).

CASE STUDY

Andy, 60, laryngeal cancer survivor

Recognising the value of your new role

Andy had his voice box removed during treatment. He had to give up work as a chef, and felt that not only had he lost his role as his family's provider, but he had also lost his role as the one who stands up for the family. Andy described to me how he had always been protective of his family, sometimes getting into arguments or even fights if he felt people were threatening his loved ones.

He had also been a sociable and lively member of his local fishing group. Since his cancer he was no longer going to the river with his mates. He was relying on his wife to speak on his behalf at home. He was avoiding other people.

I encouraged Andy to look more deeply at what his family actually valued about him. He looked back at the times he felt he had 'stood up' for his family and realised that sometimes it had

→

actually made things worse (he remembered, for instance, arguing with his son's teacher – and then his son not wanting to go to school any more). He was also amazed when he asked his children what they felt about him having lost his job. They all said they were sorry for him but they enjoyed having him around at home more. They didn't mind having less money as they were starting to earn their own. And they told him they didn't feel embarrassed walking down the street any more, because they knew, now, that they wouldn't have to apologise to neighbours for one of their dad's rants.

Andy gradually realised that now he was home more, he was helping his family in other ways. He helped his daughter to think through how to manage a difficult situation with her boss. He cooked for his wife. He was there for his son during stressful exams. Andy became more aware of all the ways he interacts with, and supports his family. He was devastated to lose his job and his voice, but he began to recognise that providing for his family went way beyond money or physical strength.

By keeping a record of what he actually did, Andy became much more aware of the other things he achieved. He was older, wiser and (on the whole!) more mature than his kids and they sought him out for advice and, at times, comfort. He had the time to think about their concerns and help them through their difficult patches. He couldn't buy expensive gifts for his wife, but he could still treat her: a tasty packed lunch; a foot massage when she got in from work. Outside the family, it was difficult to be in a group – his artificial voice box made him self-conscious and it was hard to hear in a noisy environment. But he worked out ways of explaining (or joking away) this change and he asked one or two friends round to his home, where he felt more comfortable. Andy discovered that his friends still wanted his opinions and his jokes

→

(even the awful ones). By becoming aware of all these lower-key 'roles' he fulfilled, Andy built up his confidence. He gradually returned to the river and fishing. He'd found a way to adjust to the new (and at times improved) Andy.

Challenge your thoughts

Your thoughts make a huge difference to your self-esteem. But your thoughts are just your interpretation of events – they aren't a straightforward reflection of reality. Think about this for a moment. You probably know at least one clever, competent and attractive person who feels they're just not good enough. How we interpret our lives often just isn't 'reality'.

Most of us are particularly good at having unrealistic and unhelpful thoughts when it comes to body image and self-esteem. And, after cancer, people often fall into a set of common 'thought traps'. If you've been reading this book chapter by chapter, you'll know a lot about thought traps by now (if not, see pages 17–19). You could well be sick of them. But grit your teeth and keep reading because spotting your thought traps is completely central if you are to boost your self-esteem and improve how you see your own body.

COMMON BODY IMAGE AND SELF-ESTEEM 'THOUGHT TRAPS'

We all fall into unhelpful ways of thinking sometimes. The key is to recognise when you're doing it – then you can change it.

How often do you fall into these traps?

- **Mind reading**: 'My family are struggling now that I don't work'; 'They are looking at me and thinking I'm ugly'.

- **Minimising**: 'Yeah, I made lunch, but I used to do ten times as much in a day'; 'OK, so I've started to work on my weight but it will never make the scars go'.

- **Blaming yourself**: 'If only I was stronger I could stop people around me worrying'; 'If I had worn an ice cap during chemo maybe I wouldn't have lost all my hair'.

- **Double standards/harsh or unrealistic expectations of yourself**: 'I shouldn't cry'; 'It's so silly to worry about my appearance, I should just be grateful that I am alive'.

- **Emotional reasoning**: 'Because I feel useless, I am useless; I feel ugly so I am ugly'.

EXERCISE

The case for the defence

Here are three ways to tackle your thought traps:

1. **Look back at the dig deeper exercise** (on pages 125–6). Knowing more about yourself will help you to challenge some of your thought traps. Now, try to identify one of your common thought traps, using the list above or on pages 18–19. Try to argue against it, by saying 'Yes … and' (or a 'Hold on, but what about …'). For example (Thought trap: Minimising), 'I made lunch, but I used to do ten times as much in a day'. Your defence: **'Yes … and** … I've had cancer. I've got through six months of chemo; I'm struggling with fatigue and the side effects of ongoing medication. It's something that I got up and made lunch. That took determination.'

2. **Use your achievement log book to provide clear evidence for the defence**. For instance (Thought trap: Harsh

expectations), 'I'm useless, I get nothing done'. Your defence, taken from your log book, **'Hold on . . . but what about** the shopping? I got all the way to the grocery shop and back today, and now I have something for dinner.'

3. **Ask 'What am I not?'** You might also want to try coming at this from a different angle. Think, for a bit, about personality traits that you find unpleasant/unappealing and which you know are not part of your character. For instance, selfishness, cruelty, rudeness, aggression, impatience, arrogance, indecisiveness, lack of assertiveness, over-indulgence – whatever is meaningful for you. Then either think about or, if possible, write down: 'I am not (fill in the characteristic) because . . .' For example you might write: 'I am not rude because I always treat people politely and with respect'. This is a bit of a different approach, but it can really help you to get some perspective on yourself.

TACKLING THOUGHT TRAPS

Here are some other questions to ask yourself when you notice an unhelpful thought popping into your head:

1. What am I actually achieving each day?

2. Am I undermining or ignoring things I've done?

3. Are my expectations (of myself/others/this situation) reasonable?

4. What would I say to a friend in a similar situation?

5. If someone else was saying this to me, would I accept it, or would I challenge them? ('Actually, I'm not hopeless at

everything, I'm just finding it difficult to get back to work – but I'm managing my housework, I'm building up my fitness.')

6. Am I treating a thought as if it was a fact?

7. How do I know that the other person/people think this?

Rewards – and why they matter

If you have ever watched a child learn something new, you'll know how powerful a reward can be – whether it's a treat or an admiring round of applause from a doting granny. Think about a toddler who is just learning to walk. He'll get cheered and clapped when he clambers to his feet. His first steps will be greeted with wild excitement, smiles and laughter – possibly even a chocolate button and flashbulbs. If he falls down, he'll be dusted off, and encouraged to try again. This is our basic model of learning. It's deeply embedded in our minds, whether we realise it or not.

Sadly, our ability to reward ourselves tends to get lost as we grow up, particularly if our self-esteem isn't high. Learning to reward yourself is vital in building up your self-esteem. It's pretty basic – you'll want to repeat actions and thoughts if they are associated with something nice.

WAYS TO REWARD YOURSELF

1. **Thoughts and statements:** The most important rewards are free. They are the kind and supportive things you can say to yourself when something has been tough. They are also the exciting, stimulating and encouraging things you think when you've achieved something. If saying these things to yourself doesn't come readily, try writing a list

of some simple, rewarding things you could say to yourself ('You did it!', 'Great work', 'You are on track', 'Practice makes perfect', 'That was an excellent effort'). Remember that learning toddler: if he hears the encouragement enough, it will become part of the way he thinks about himself. He'll use those thoughts and statements to motivate himself for the rest of his life. Now you probably won't get the cheering crowds – as an adult it's usually up to you to keep yourself going. But think about what it does to your self-esteem when you say to yourself: 'That was hopeless, you didn't manage what you set out to achieve, you'll never amount to anything!' Compare that feeling with how you feel if you say to yourself: 'OK, you made a start, you're on the way. It was an effort, but you're further on than you were this morning. Well done – more tomorrow.' It's pretty obvious which one will keep you motivated to face the challenges of the next day, week or month.

2. **Treats**: Only you can know what your idea of a treat is, but anything will do as long as you like it, whether it's a bunch of roses, a new magazine, a phone call to a friend, a bar of chocolate, a day off washing up, a walk in the park, a trip to bowling, a bet on the horses ... It just has to be something relatively easy, that you enjoy.

TIP ▶

REMIND YOURSELF WHY YOU'RE HAVING THE REWARD

Whatever treat you choose, make sure that when you indulge – the moment you slide into the bath, open the magazine or sink your teeth into the chocolate, you actually remind yourself why you deserve this. What goal or achievement are you celebrating? Also, remember to vary your treats – the same one gets boring, even if you love it in theory.

Just do it . . .

Rewarding yourself might not come easy. You'll probably feel self-conscious, perhaps a bit guilty. But it really is vital to do this. There is solid scientific evidence to show that rewards will help you to change the way you think about yourself. So, when it comes to building self-esteem, if you only try only one thing from this chapter, then make it this: **when you manage to think helpful thoughts or make it onto the next step of the ladder that leads you to your goal then reward yourself.**

When to get help

Feeling uncertain about yourself, dissatisfied with your body and generally low are all very natural after finishing cancer treatment. But this is such a difficult thing to go through, and if it goes on for too long it can really damage your quality of life. Don't suffer in silence. Give yourself time and try not to expect too much too soon, but also do be aware that there's help out there. If your thoughts about your body become extreme and if you find yourself thinking about harming yourself talk to your medical team, your GP or call a cancer helpline or Samaritans straight away.

Medical teams may be able to tackle some body image issues – offering colostomy reversals (where possible), breast reconstruction or plastic surgery. Further surgery is rarely a perfect solution. It does need careful consideration and doesn't always address the emotional side of poor body image or low self-esteem, but it can help some people to feel better about themselves.

Making an appointment with a counsellor (via your GP) or seeing staff at your local cancer support service can also help you to process what you've been through, and find a way forward. Sometimes, expert support is what you need most of all.

Self-esteem and body image are complicated things. But they really are important if you are to get your life back on track – cope with the changes you've been through, and heal. It isn't self-indulgent to think about any of this – it's necessary. If it helps, then you could always think of this as a gift to other people: if you feel stronger, more confident and more reconciled to your new self, then your loved ones, colleagues and friends will reap the benefit too.

Family, friends and carers: How you can help someone with low self-esteem

Knowing what to say or how to help someone whose self-esteem or body image has taken a big knock can be a real challenge. Changing the way you see yourself takes time and effort. It's a very personal process that's hard to speed up. But other people can definitely help.

The suggestions in Chapter 2: Depression and Low Mood for supporting someone who is depressed are all generally relevant here (see pages 80–2). The issues aren't exactly the same but patience, trying not to get into debates, giving clear evidence to counter their unhelpful thoughts and looking at your own expectations are all useful ways to help.

The following tips are also particularly relevant when you're supporting a person whose body image or self-esteem has been damaged.

COPING STRATEGY

Five ways to help someone whose body image or self-esteem is damaged

1. **Show them they're valued.** Using words and actions, demonstrate that you want to be with that person, or value their opinion (if you do). Things like saying you are pleased to see them when you get in from work, arranging a date night, asking their opinion on a thorny issue in the office are all helpful.

2. **Be honest.** A person with low self-esteem will have a strong insincerity radar. If you are in a bad mood, explain why or they are likely to assume it is something to do with them. If it is to do with them, then focus your comment on the particular thing they did, on that specific day/at that moment, rather than anything sweeping or general. For example, instead of global statements like 'You're always miserable' or 'You never want to go out', try something more 'local', for instance: 'I wish you had come out to walk the dog with me this evening.'

3. **Notice what they do and comment on it.** Remember the baby learning to walk? If he hadn't got the round of applause he probably would have flopped back onto his bottom for a few more months. Again, don't be insincere or over the top: a quick comment when you see them achieving something will be noticed.

4. **Ask if they need any particular help or support from you.** Then ask again – once is rarely enough. But only do this when you really are willing to help. Offering help, then giving the impression that it's a burden, will be counter-productive. A good approach is to support the person as they tackle exercises from this chapter (or anything in this book). Showing genuine interest in them and their progress

(or, at times, their setbacks) will help a lot. You could start by reading the rest of this book yourself if you haven't already.

5. **Help them to think constructively**. People with low self-esteem or who are struggling with their body image often ask for reassurance – sometimes repeatedly. This can be irritating, or worrying, or just plain repetitive, and it often doesn't actually do much good. You have to judge for yourself how much reassurance your loved one/friend really needs from you, but sometimes, instead of automatically responding to a 'Do you still love me?' with 'Of course I do' you could try saying: 'I wonder what you think? Do you think I love you? What do you think I love about you?' Of course, pick the right time, and say it in a supportive way, then back it up with very clear 'evidence' of just how much you love them and why. But doing this means that they have to stop and think for themselves for a moment – they almost have to answer their own question. This stops the exchange from becoming automatic and not terribly productive. It turns it into something more thoughtful that helps them to build up a good picture of themselves.

CHAPTER FIVE

RELATIONSHIPS AND SEX

> 6 I know it was Tyra who was coping with the cancer. But I felt like I'd been hit by a tornado. I knew I was meant to be strong for her but I didn't know how: my whole world had been turned upside down. 9

JACK, BOYFRIEND OF TYRA, 34, BRAIN CANCER SURVIVOR

How cancer changes relationships

You don't have to be a psychologist to recognise that your experience of cancer affects other people too. Your partner, family, friends and colleagues – they've all been through something huge with you. Of course, it's you who has gone through the trauma of actual diagnosis and treatment. But the truth is that the people close to you – people who care about you – have faced unsettling changes too, both emotional and practical.

Your cancer may have caused them to take a long, hard look at their beliefs; about the people they love, about the world around them. Their life will have been shaken up too. All this means that when it comes to 'getting back on track' things can get pretty complicated.

Changes to relationships during treatment

During treatment, family, friends and communities tend to kick into action (though of course this doesn't always happen!). They tend to become practical and protective. There is, after all, a lot to get done at this stage – they can gather information, let people know what's happening, get you to and from hospital appointments, arrange care for children or elderly relatives, cook, clean, manage the medication – the list seems endless.

This can feel like a lifeline. 'My colleagues at work drew up a rota for who would take me to my hospital appointments and visit me during my admissions,' says Rosa, 52, breast cancer survivor. 'They also left me homemade meals to put into the microwave for dinner, and telephoned me every night to check I was OK. I never felt alone. I was so supported.'

But while all this is going on, roles are often disrupted. The person who does the school run, cooking or housework might have to change. Your partner might take time off work to nurse you. You might move back in with your parents. The office has to function without its manager. The local football club loses its referee.

FAITH

If you have a religious or spiritual faith, this might change too. Your faith may have been challenged by your experience with cancer. Maybe you're now struggling to find the support you need from your spiritual leader or your religious texts. Or, perhaps it's the opposite. Perhaps your faith feels strengthened – you find solace in prayer, reading, talking or being in your place of worship. Some people even develop a faith they didn't have before, or explore new religions or spiritual paths that sustain them through the storm of cancer. Either way, there can be any number of changes to your faith after cancer and they can be profound – life altering even.

Not rocking the boat

While all this is happening, people tend to swallow their resentments and objections. They put up with things they wouldn't normally accept. They don't want to rock that already very shaky boat. And such changes might all be perfectly reasonable during the storm of diagnosis and treatment. Everyone is feeling the pressure together. Nobody wants to whip up the waves any more. Everyone wants to do their bit.

'During treatment, I felt dependent on my husband, Keith,' says Mary, 71, ovarian cancer survivor. 'He was doing so much for me. It seemed unreasonable to ask him to turn off his folk music. I've always hated folk – in the past I could just move away. But when I was in bed, I'd hear him whistling along to it in the kitchen, and I wanted to scream. But I couldn't because I knew his music was keeping him sane.'

Then, when treatment ends, and your medical team lifeboat sails off into the sunset, everything is supposed to be 'normal' again.

But it isn't.

Roles have changed. There has been a lot of worry and stress and strain and pressure – and avoidance. Is there any surprise that relationships can get tricky?

This can feel very lonely. Sometimes one of the toughest aspects of finishing treatment is the sense of not quite having made it 'back' to safety: it's as if your 'boat' has washed up on the beach – not in the safety of the harbour. You can see all the people on shore waving at you, and calling you back, but you can't quite get to them.

'I can be in a busy office at work, surrounded by my family at home, lying in the arms of my wife at night, and I've never felt more lonely,' says George, 49, rectal cancer survivor.

You are facing the huge task of rebuilding and mending your boat. But so are your family and friends. And this is the exact point where relationships start to feel the strain and problems crop up.

Couples after cancer: From rock to rocky

It is extremely common for people to talk about their partner being 'a rock' throughout cancer treatment. But when treatment ends, there can be misunderstandings and conflicts. A lot of couples start to feel emotionally and physically distant.

'Jack was amazing through my treatment,' says Tyra, 34, brain cancer survivor. 'He made me laugh through my tears, he was a breath of fresh air after my anxious parents and he got really involved in my care. But now that I'm better it feels hard to get that intimacy and closeness back. We're living together again but we seem to spend more time arguing about who last cleaned the bathroom than talking about what is really important in life.'

COMMON RELATIONSHIP PROBLEMS AFTER CANCER

Relationship problems – not just in couples, but among families, friends and colleagues – tend to have common themes post-cancer. Here are the main ones:

Your expectations of yourself

- **Expecting too much of yourself:** 'I have turned into such a nasty person. I used to be so calm and patient but now the tiniest thing can make me fly off the handle.'

- **Unrealistic time pressures:** 'I should be over this by now. I don't understand why I don't feel able to get back to doing the things we used to enjoy, like a day at the seaside or an event at the village hall.'

Other people's expectations of you

- **Over-protectiveness**: 'I'm building up my strength again through regular exercise but my partner keeps saying that I am doing too much and will make myself ill again.'

- **Pressure to be 'normal' again**: 'My boss calls every day to ask when I am going back to work. It's only been a month and I don't feel ready.'

- **Unrealistic expectations**: 'I've only finished treatment a week ago and already it's as if my cancer had never happened: my wife and kids have dumped everything straight back on me.'

Changed roles

- **I want my life back!** 'My husband is much more involved in the lives of the children now. He doesn't want to give up doing the school run, but I see that as my role and I want it back.'

- **I've been pushed out**: 'My deputy took on lots of my work while I was off sick, but now I'm back he wants to keep doing my job. Our boss seems to agree; he keeps saying I should take things easy and see what new role comes up.'

Sleeping volcanoes

- 'My husband thinks he was Florence Nightingale when I was ill. He thinks that that gives him the right to control me now; well, it doesn't. We are having big fights, and we never used to.' (If you store up resentments or anxieties they tend to fester. And when they finally blow, they can be huge.)

What to do about these problems

First, what not to do …

Avoidance and why it won't work

Yes, we're back there again. Avoidance never works. But it can be really difficult to talk honestly with people after treatment, and it can feel much easier to just 'let it go'. You've got used to skirting over difficult subjects, papering the cracks and keeping the peace because nobody wants more stress during cancer. The only problem is that it doesn't work any more. There are tensions, misunderstandings and resentments. And it's hard to know how to broach these when you're used to burying them in silence.

It might feel ungrateful to be critical, when people have done so much to help. 'My friends were so kind to me,' says Gregor, 56, mouth cancer survivor. 'But I don't know how to tell them that I don't need so much help now. In fact, I'd really like to be left alone a bit.'

COPING STRATEGY

How to rebuild relationships after cancer

Step 1: Give yourself time

Many of the problems that arise in couples, families and between friends post-cancer come down to unrealistic or unclear expectations. Nobody can tell you how long it's going to take to recover. Everyone is different. But one thing's certain: the idea that people just bounce back instantly after cancer is a myth. Absolutely everybody needs some time to adjust. Often it's a question of working out your own way of doing this.

Step 2: Get information (be specific)

If you ask your healthcare team 'When will my relationships feel normal again?', they'll say we're all individuals and everyone responds to cancer recovery in their own way, so it's impossible to predict. But if you say: 'My boss is expecting me back at work a month after treatment — is this realistic?' or 'I told my mother I want to go back to rugby training, but she doesn't think I'm up to it', you'll probably get a very different answer.

Ask your team what, in their experience, is the average recovery time for specific physical activities and tasks. Ask them about the faster and slower recovery times, too. You may get more useful information and then you will be able to use this, when talking to friends, family or your partner about recovery expectations.

Step 3: Get support

If you are feeling very alone, even though you may be surrounded by other people, it can really help to talk to someone else who has been through a similar situation. It can be reassuring to know that you're not the only one to have felt this way. Knowing that others have been through similar experiences can help you to feel connected. It can also give you hope that you will rebuild your relationships. It's possible that right now what you need most is support from another cancer survivor (via a local support group or from someone you know — even if you're not particularly close to them already).

This worked really well for Jamal, 35, testicular cancer survivor. 'My father's friend wrote to me after my treatment finished and told me that he too had had testicular cancer in his 30s,' he says. 'He said that if I ever wanted to talk to him he would be happy to meet up. At my lowest moment my partner forced me to call him. It was the best thing I did. It was like he could finish my sentences for me – he knew what I was going through and I didn't feel so alone any more.'

If you aren't someone who enjoys too much talking, there are other resources too: this book should at least help you to know that you're not alone, and if you go online to a cancer support organisation (or put yourself on their mailing lists) you'll hear about other people's stories even if you don't want to share your own. Sometimes you just need personal anecdotes that will let you know that you're not the only one feeling as you do.

Step 4: Communicate

Yes, that dreaded c-word. When a relationship is under strain, and an 'expert' tells you to **communicate**, it's like a nurse lunging at you with a huge syringe shouting 'relax!'

But, if you are still shaken up by cancer – and you may be, months or even years later – you are probably still in 'protective' mode: not really talking about difficult things, not wanting to rock the boat, just knuckling down and getting on with it. This can make communication in relationships very difficult indeed.

You, and people close to you, might be quite confused about what you actually feel right now. The notion of 'dredging it all up' can seem scary. 'It's just too hard to talk about our feelings about the cancer,' says Annabel, 68, bowel cancer survivor. 'If we tried we'd just open the floodgates so it is better just talking about day-to-day stuff.'

A lot of people also worry that talking is just going to stress them out – and after everything they've been through more stress is the last thing they need. But if you don't communicate, it can soon feel that you are living on different planets. This is stressful. Indeed, over time, it can be much more stressful than biting the bullet and talking about how you feel.

CASE STUDY

Dan, 53, oesophageal cancer survivor

Recovery time

Dan, a civil servant, kept in contact with work throughout his cancer treatment. He returned to work as soon as he could after treatment ended (three weeks in his case). He seemed to be coping. But two years later he found himself feeling very low. His marriage was under strain. He became quite depressed. And it was at this point that he realised that he needed to take some time out.

Dan was well supported by his occupational health department and GP, and was able to take six weeks off work. He had some counselling with me, but mostly he just spent this time with his wife, children and their new grandchild. He also recognised that he needed time alone – and his family respected and encouraged this. Dan surprised himself, having never been religious, by walking into his local church one day. It felt like a peaceful place where he could try to think about everything he'd been through. The vicar approached, and accepted that Dan was not seeking religious guidance. Instead, he simply sat near him for a while, offering silent companionship and support. Dan badly needed time to process what he and his family had all been through. He had thought he could do it all and just bounce back, but it caught up with him in the end. 'I didn't realise it, but there was a lot I'd never dealt with,' he said. 'I realised how badly I just needed space, a kind of silent refuge.'

Different worlds

Tyra's been through so much and still has so far to go, I don't feel as if it is fair to burden her with the news that my job is under threat and my boss is talking about relocating to Wales,' says Jack, boyfriend of Tyra.

'I had no idea why Jack wasn't talking to me,' says Tyra. 'I could tell something was on his mind, but it's as if he doesn't feel we have a two-way relationship any more. He seems to think it is now all about him supporting me. It's like he doesn't trust me.'

What communication actually means

In an ideal world:

- you talk clearly about each person's perspective
- you listen to all points of view
- you negotiate an agreed way forward.

Obviously, it's rarely that simple. This is why it can help to have a structure for your talking. If you have a structure, you won't 'open the floodgates' or whip up too much emotion. And even if it does feel stressful, at times, remember that **stress will not make the cancer come back** (see page 60).

Talking about cancer and the emotions associated with it is not going to affect your medical outcome. But it might well distinctly improve the quality of life – for everyone concerned.

... And repeat

People often think that communication means having the 'big talk' and then – that's it – you're done, right?

Sadly, no. It rarely works like this. It is particularly the case with couples. With couples, sometimes one partner will feel, after the 'big talk' that it's done and dusted but the other really needs to keep talking. And talking. And talking.

'We talked together once about our fears that the cancer might come back and that seems to have been enough for Eve,' says Darius, 63, kidney cancer survivor. 'But it isn't for me. I keep trying to talk to her about it but I just get told that we've said enough and what else can we say? I just feel selfish, bringing it up.'

It often works this way with reassurance too – one partner might need a lot of it, repeatedly. 'I've told her that I love her just as much as I did before her cancer,' says Steve, husband of Jan, 57, breast cancer survivor. 'So I don't understand why she wants me to say it over and over again.'

Cancer can leave long-lasting scars – not just physical ones. And the only way to heal these scars, within relationships, is to talk, sometimes a lot.

How to talk to each other

EXERCISE

Talk time

If – as a couple or family – you go to see a therapist, there are safe boundaries. You all know why you're there, you have a counsellor to guide you, you stick to a time limit, you are in a neutral place, there are rules about taking it in turns to speak, listening to the other person, and making sure each of you expresses yourself so that on the whole the session is kept relatively controlled. But you don't necessarily need a therapist to communicate effectively with lovers, family, friends or colleagues. You can instead borrow some of the tricks of the trade to create a safe and contained way to talk.

Try setting up a regular 'talk time' with clear ground rules. Fix a regular slot where you will get together and talk about how things are going. This could be Sunday evening for a family review of the week, a monthly support/appraisal session at work, or a daily time slot, set aside just for talking to your partner.

The rules of talk time

1. **Set clear boundaries**. Be clear that the idea behind this 'session' is to focus on how people are actually feeling. Everyone gets a say, and everyone is expected to listen.

2. **Find a neutral place** – maybe outside your home, or work-place. At the very least, if you can physically move out of a room at the end of the 'talk time' it is much easier to draw a line under it, and get on with your day.

3. **Set a time limit and stick to it**. If you are going over the time limit: don't. Stop and arrange another session. It can be overwhelming to leave these talk times open-ended. (See Tip below.)

4. **Structure it your way** – you'll know what works for you – maybe it will help if you set a brief agenda, or have a short time, a minute or two each, where each person gets a chance to speak without being interrupted. It can help to set aside some time for negotiation (discussing how any changes can work) or goal setting (agreeing what you're all aiming to achieve). Make sure, at your next talk time, that you include a time where you look over the progress you've made. It sounds formal, particularly in a relation-ship or family, but these rules can work wonders. Without them, it can feel like chaos.

5. **Avoid interruptions**. Turn phones off and don't answer the

front door. Unless the house is burning down, talk time is sacred.

6. **Find a good way to end.** Maybe one person could sum up what's been said, or you could end with a 'to do' list. If it's your partner or family you're talking to, you could move on to something you all like doing together (Your favourite TV show? Walking the dog together? A Wii game?).

TIP ▶

If all this talking sounds really gruesome to you, then it's fine to set a really short talk time limit to begin with – even just five or ten minutes of brief talking is a useful starting point.

CASE STUDY

Tyra, 34, brain cancer survivor

Talk time

Tyra and her partner Jack were referred to me by their GP when they said they needed some relationship support after her brain cancer.

We used 'talk time' to help them communicate better. They liked the idea of drawing up an agenda, and they decided that giving Jack some time to talk about his experience of Tyra's cancer was the starting point.

Tyra let him talk. She didn't interrupt him and she listened very carefully. He spoke almost non-stop for half an hour. Then Tyra talked, not about her experiences, but about her response to what Jack had said. →

It was very moving for them both: he'd never told her how frightened he'd been, or how vulnerable he'd felt. She admitted that she'd hardly thought about Jack's feelings – he was a solid support, and she'd been far more worried about what her parents were feeling.

They only had two meetings with me. After their first meeting they set up a weekly 'talk time' on a Thursday night in their local Italian restaurant. They structured each of these evenings to address a different concern, including renegotiating their roles at home, talking about their hopes (and fears) for the future, and setting some goals.

Jack was able to tell Tyra about his work problems and the possibility of a move to Wales, and was amazed to discover that she quite liked the idea of relocating. Tyra was able to tell Jack how much she wanted to have children but how anxious she was about what treatment might have done to her fertility. Jack told her that he did want children, but he wanted to be with her whether they had children or not. They arranged to go flat hunting in Cardiff, talk to Tyra's consultant about fertility, and to book a holiday.

At our second meeting I pointed out that they'd been having problems negotiating the household tasks. They decided to take a structured approach to this, too: they drew up a rota and talked about their different standards of cleanliness.

Jack and Tyra didn't feel they needed any more appointments with me. They sent me their wedding pictures a year later. Of course, not everyone will find their relationship issues this straightforward to resolve – not by any means. But, taking a structured approach to communication is almost always an excellent place to start.

Talking to children

When talking to children about your cancer it's important to realise that you may have to go over and over things. As children develop, their understanding of cancer will develop too. They are likely to need to talk about what happened to you at every stage of their development. Even if you thought the issue was ancient history, it might not be for them.

There are books and leaflets that can help you to talk to children (you may have seen these during treatment). These are fine, but use your own instincts too – it's your cancer, and your children. You probably have the best idea of how to support them.

Talking to children about cancer (even when it is in the past) can be really difficult and upsetting. Often, it looks as if the children don't want or need to talk. But remember what sponges children are – they'll suck up every little bit of overheard conversation, they'll pick up on tiny facial expressions, they'll get information from outside sources – and they'll usually come to their own, possibly completely inaccurate, conclusion about what's happening to you. Establishing a regular talk time can help to keep your children informed and reassured (see Resources for further advice on talking to children).

Talking to your boss

'Talk time' works well with your boss too. It is usually better to arrange a meeting, and be clear about what you are going to discuss, than just to grab a quick word over the water cooler, and hope you got your point across. Decisions about your return to work or any adjustments you need, or how you're doing, need thoughtful consideration, not instant solutions. You and your boss both need time to consider and plan what you want to say and what strategies are needed. Communication needs to be ongoing, too, because what you need and what you can do will change. As a rule make sure that whenever one meeting is coming to an end, you set a date for the next one. If you happen to be the boss, the same rules apply when talking to your team or colleagues. You're likely to need some adjustments to your work environment. You may require some extra help. It's really vital to be clear about what you need.

People often find it helpful to get an advocate to come with them when they are trying to communicate at work. This sounds official and complicated, but in fact just means you have someone with you who can speak for you if and when you find it difficult. In an ideal world, we'd all speak up for ourselves but there are times – and cancer is one of them – when we might need a little help from our friends.

Dan, oesophageal cancer survivor (see page 146), felt a lot more confident talking to his boss after his six weeks off, with his occupational health adviser alongside him. Dan could update his boss on his progress, and ask for additional support, but the occupational health adviser was able to discuss legal rights and frameworks that Dan didn't feel confident (or comfortable) talking about.

COUPLES AND FAMILIES: OTHER THINGS TO TRY

- **Change your environment or routine.** If talk time sounds like hell to you (or to one of you) then you might prefer something less structured. Communication can be tricky if you are stuck in a rut. But often, just changing your routines can make it suddenly easier to talk.

- **Getting away for a bit.** Getting out of your home and your usual routines – a holiday, a long weekend away, even a meal out – can encourage communication just because the venue's different. Of course, cancer may have left you feeling physically and financially low. But you don't have to cruise the Caribbean.

- **Small changes work too**. Turn off the TV for the evening, take a stroll round a park you don't know well, cook something unusual together, get out an old board game or suggest a trip to a pub that's not your local.

Rewards

Rewards can be a great confidence boost when you are making difficult changes together (see page 132 for why rewards and treats are vital). Rewarding your progress doesn't just work for the things you do on your own. The principle applies to couples, families and friendships too.

You have all been through a shocking and extreme situation. Relationships need nourishment at the best of times, and after some of the worst times they need serious tender loving care. But somehow, after cancer, people end up focusing on the little niggles and stresses (like cleaning the bathroom, in the case of Jack and Tyra). These niggles and stresses are the topsoil of any relationship: they're the visible, sometimes bumpy, sometimes dry earth you can see on the flower bed. But they aren't the rich, deep, nurturing soil under the surface – the soil that allows a relationship to put down its roots and really blossom. To make any relationship work, you need fun, happy, shared times together too. It isn't selfish or spoilt to treat yourself as a couple, a family, a friendship: it's completely essential (you need to feed those relationship roots). Again, it might help to make a list of things you enjoy doing together – it can be as simple as a takeaway, a foot massage or an old-fashioned game of Monopoly.

> **TIP▶**
>
> ### KNOW WHEN TO SHUT UP
>
> OK, so, for pages now you've been reading about nothing but talk, talk, talk. You'll no doubt be relieved to hear that there are moments when the best-laid talking plans just don't work. The Sunday night family review might clash with a birthday party or a favourite film. Or you might just get to the end of an exhausting weekend and know that you aren't going to be able to discuss your feelings without screaming at each other. This is OK. You don't need to talk about this, or analyse it in depth. It is only not OK if it keeps happening. That's avoidance and (yes, you've read this before) avoidance is never a good thing. But once in a while when someone really doesn't feel like talking that's fine. Set a new time or date and let the old one pass.

Thought traps

It is not always the talking that can be tricky in relationships. Your thoughts can make things difficult, too. Here are some very common relationship thought traps. If you become aware of these then you can change them into more helpful ways of thinking. This, in turn, will have a direct impact on your relationship. How many on this list are familiar to you?

- **Mind reading**: 'She thinks I'm weak'; 'This is such a burden for him.'

- **Fortune telling**: 'We never used to bicker like this; we're going to split up'; 'She'll never agree to this idea.'

- **'All or nothing' thinking**: 'If we don't sort out our difficulties now we never will'; 'I must be cheerful all the time otherwise my friends will panic.'

- **Thinking the worst**: 'If I tell him how I feel he's going to leave me'; 'If I don't express myself clearly I'll never be understood.'

- **Harsh or unrealistic expectations**: 'I should be able to cope with this without banging on about my feelings'; 'I shouldn't take up any more of my boss's time.'

- **Ignoring the positives**: 'We only ever talk about boring stuff'; 'They say they want me back at work but they have to say that, don't they?'

- **Labelling/blaming**: 'I am so weak not to be able to talk about this'; 'He is so selfish.'

COPING STRATEGY

How to change your thoughts

Try to notice what thoughts are running through your head when you are thinking about your relationships and how you communicate.

1. **Write down these thoughts**: It's only when you see them written down that you can see the reality of what you're actually saying to yourself. Sometimes it's amazing how harsh we can be on ourselves and also others.

2. **Identify your thought traps**: Look at the ones listed above. Do any apply to you? In particular, try to spot when you're making big, sweeping comments to yourself, when the reality isn't quite so dramatic. For instance, do you really only **ever** talk about boring stuff? Do you have to be cheerful **all** the time?

TIP▶

ARGUE BACK

Examine the things you are saying in your head – about yourself and about other people. Now, imagine if it was someone you don't know very well saying that to you. Would you agree with them, or might you challenge them? For example, if someone said to you that you or your partner was really lazy/stupid/selfish etc., how would you respond? No doubt you'd tell them where to get off. So, why do you have a different rule for yourself?

Accepting change

The storm of cancer may have changed your family or relationships. It has probably left some damage, washed up a bit of flotsam and jetsam, maybe broken a few things along the way. But perhaps it also uncovered some treasures too. Your life and relationships might look different now, but different does not automatically mean worse. It may take some time to explore and get used to this new way of being with your friends, colleagues, partner and family – particularly as it's a change you didn't ask for let alone want – but you've weathered a storm together, and that's worth a lot. Sometimes, the real trick is just learning to accept that it's changed.

Sexual relationships

Sex during treatment

Let's face it, there probably wasn't any. During treatment, you may have been too ill to contemplate any form of sexual activity, and your partner may well have been too stressed and protective to have much in the way of a sex drive either.

Cancer can directly affect the sexual organs and libido. Major surgical interventions of any sort will prevent sexual activity for some time. Pain or side effects such as pins and needles or nausea can make touching or holding uncomfortable. Night-time symptoms – insomnia, temperature changes, night sweats, the need to pee, nausea and vomiting – mean that couples often end up sleeping in separate beds.

All of this does not just mean that it's only sex that is off the agenda. It often means that any kind of physical intimacy – cuddling, touching, kissing – goes out the window too. Cancer can be incredibly distancing for a couple. And it can make sex feel like a huge hurdle when you are 'supposed' to be picking up where you left off.

Sex after cancer treatment

You wouldn't think it, from the lack of discussion on the subject, but it is extraordinarily common to have difficulties with sex after cancer.

'My husband and I had been having a very good sex life, much better than when we had been bringing up our young children,' says Barbara, 56, a breast cancer survivor. 'That's why it's so upsetting that it's all stopped now. We tried, but it was awkward and uncomfortable and we've just given up. I know that we are both unhappy about it but I guess that is just the way it is after cancer.'

With cancers that have affected the sexual organs – gynaecological, breast, prostate and testicular cancers, for instance – the effect on your sex life is obvious. Treatments such as hormonal therapy, surgery or radiotherapy can cause vaginal tightening, dryness and reduced sex drive, while surgery and radiotherapy, in testicular and prostate cancers, can affect erectile function and libido. But even in the more obvious cases, people often underestimate the impact of a disrupted sex life. Most of all, they avoid discussing it.

For the partner of a cancer survivor, the issues can be particularly tricky – and again, they're hardly ever talked about. Many people are worried that they will hurt their partner, who has obviously 'suffered enough'. They also worry that they are imposing their own desires and needs when their partner is not interested. They sometimes are frightened of the physical changes to their partner, and some people even worry that having sex could make them catch the cancer (it can't), or could trigger it again in their partner (it won't!).

Even medical teams can find this hard to tackle. Some medical staff may feel uncomfortable asking a patient about their sexual function – and many patients won't want to ask about it. There tends to be a lack of practical information and advice about when and how to resume sex. You might wonder whether it's appropriate to talk about this at all. A wall of silence develops.

There may also be unrealistic expectations thrown into the mix: often people assume that they'll just pick up where they left off when it comes to sex. They are then flummoxed to find that it's not that straightforward. Or, they assume the opposite – that their sex life is over for good.

Thinking about sex

Cancer does not just affect your sex drive and bodily functions. It can affect your body image and self-esteem too (see Chapter 4: Self-esteem and Body Image). These directly affect your sex life.

Not surprisingly, many of those unhelpful thought traps then kick in. Here are some common ones, when it comes to sex:

- **Mind reading**: 'He'll hate having to look at my mastectomy site.'

- **Fortune telling**: 'Our relationship is going to break down if we can't have penetrative sex.'
- **Unrealistic/unhelpful expectations**: 'I should be feeling good about my body. It got through cancer. I should love it.'
- **Ignoring the positives**: 'She says she loves me just as much as before but she's just being kind.'

CASE STUDY

Barbara, 56, breast cancer survivor

Thought traps

*Barbara had fallen into several thought traps. She told me that she felt that her husband Tony no longer found her attractive (**mind reading**). Although he told her he loved her several times each day he was only doing that because he was in the habit of saying it (**ignoring the positives**). She worried that he might leave her (**fortune telling**) and she thought that if they didn't have sex at least once a fortnight now that her cancer was gone, then this showed that their relationship was damaged (**unrealistic/ unhelpful expectations**).*

*Tony, meanwhile, had developed a few thought traps of his own. He didn't think Barbara liked him touching her (**mind reading**). He was frightened that she had stopped loving him (**thinking the worst**). He felt that it was not for him to bring up the topic of sex, since it was Barbara who'd been through the trauma of cancer treatment – she'd talk to him when she was ready (**unrealistic/ unhelpful expectations**).*

Looking at Barbara and Tony's thought traps you can probably see how they ended up in a vicious circle of not talking about

→

their sex life. This meant that they got more anxious about it. The pressure and expectations whenever they did try to have sex were overwhelming.

I encouraged Barbara and Tony to talk about their assumptions and expectations. They were surprised by what they learned about each other's thoughts. We then worked together to re-establish their closeness using simple, gradual steps (see page 163).

TIP▶

GO IT ALONE

In an ideal world, you'd sit down with your partner and explore these thought traps together. But if your partner is unwilling, don't just ignore all this. Even if you can't do this together, it can still help a lot to understand how your own thoughts aren't helping, and to change this. When you find yourself thinking something unhelpful, ask yourself what evidence you have that this thought really is true. This can help you work out what are unrealistic assumptions or expectations, and can help to build your confidence in yourself – even if you partner isn't involved.

How to get back in the saddle

Step 1: Tackle any physical problems

Your sex life might be disrupted by practicalities: body issues such as vaginal dryness, pain, or problems getting or maintaining an erection. Your medical team is the first port of call here. The vast majority of healthcare workers will be supportive, knowledgeable and practical if you talk to them. They will have seen it all before. There are many really effective ways to tackle post-cancer sexual problems, from vaginal lubricants or dilators, to adjusting your medication levels. Don't suffer in silence or assume that damage to your sex life is an inevitable side effect of what you've been through.

Step 2: Talk about sex

It seems obvious, but so often talking to each other about sex gets lost in all the post-cancer chaos. It can be surprisingly hard to talk about sex, even in a strong, open relationship. You may not be used to discussing it at all – it just happens (or not).

TIP▶

'SEX TALK TIME'

This may not be as exciting as it sounds – but it can help to establish some specific time where you talk about your sex life together. The same rules apply here as they do with discussing more general emotions (see 'talk time', pages 148–50). Here is an issue you could address to start with.

What do you both actually want?

There are so many automatic assumptions and myths when it comes to sex. It is worth, at the very outset, asking each other what each of you actually wants. For example, you might assume that your partner needs to have penetrative sex, when in fact what they're really desperate for is the emotional closeness of lying in bed together, hugging. Barbara, for instance, assumed that she and Tony must have fortnightly sex or it was all a disaster. But in fact, Tony didn't care how often they did it – what bothered him was that they'd become more distant in the evenings, watching different TV programmes in different rooms. This seemed to him to be a sign that their marriage was disintegrating.

How to re-establish your sex life

1. Go slow

Start by **not** having sex. Yes, really.

Sex may have become a major source of anxiety. And you may have started to avoid it, because of that anxiety.

So, take a few steps back and take away the pressure to perform. The idea is to rebuild your physical closeness before you even begin to think about actual sex. Here's how:

- **Establish a rule that you will not have sex.** Stick to that rule. Only go back to full sexual intercourse when you have worked through the other steps below and you both decide that this is what you want. For some couples it may only take a couple of weeks, while for others it may be months, and some will not get back to full penetrative sex at all (this isn't the disaster it might seem: see page 165). This does not mean that an exciting, stimulating, intimate and loving part of your relationship is out of bounds: sex is so much more than intercourse.

- **Work on building up intimacy instead** – talking to each other (and listening!), touching, stroking, showing affection, making eye contact, cuddling, kissing – no penetrative sex. Stick to the rule. These are your building blocks.

- **Set yourselves specific steps** that build up – over weeks or even months – towards penetrative sex.

EXAMPLE

The sex ladder (not quite as thrilling as it sounds)

Below is a possible list of steps on your sex ladder, building up towards penetrative sex (if that is your aim).

- Make a plan that you hold hands when going out for a walk or while watching TV.

- After a week or fortnight of this (whatever timescale you choose), move to the next step – kissing on the sofa.

- After you've done this (well, maybe not continuously) for a week or so, move to the next step: kissing in bed.

- You can add hugging, touching, foreplay, in stages: but still no penetrative sex! Even if you think you feel like it. Stick to the ban.

- Some couples find that getting to the stage where they are comfortable with mutual masturbation is a good thing to aim for. For some couples, this might be the successful end point.

- Others may then want and physically be able to move on to penetrative sex. But go through all the stages first.

CASE STUDY

Barbara, 56, breast cancer survivor

Sex ladder

Barbara and her husband Tony thought the idea of not having sex was hilarious. But they both realised it was actually a big relief when the pressure was gone. They climbed their ladder (see above) and talked a lot about their feelings for each other. And

→

they quickly discovered that while sex was important to them, what they really loved was getting back their old feelings of closeness and 'togetherness'. They quickly stopped spending their evenings 'together but apart'; they negotiated what to watch on TV and sat together. But they also watched less TV, spent time gardening and went on walks together. They looked after their grandchildren, had a trip to the cinema and even went out on a date. They chose to take two months to reach the point of having penetrative sex. The sex was emotional for them both, and they enjoyed it (even though it was a little bit awkward at the start). But it wasn't the thing they focused on any more. They felt like they were falling in love again – both of them said their sex problems had been a huge block in their relationship, making them feel distant and isolated for the first time in their thirty-two-year marriage. Getting past their difficulties helped them to reclaim so much more than their sex life.

TIP►

PENETRATION ISN'T EVERYTHING

It is important to acknowledge that cancer treatment may make full sexual intercourse for some couples very difficult. But if that's the case for you, it doesn't mean a meaningful sexual life is over. You might need to get creative – try sex toys, sexy lingerie, new techniques – but just because penetrative sex won't work any more, it doesn't mean all sexual intimacy is over.

2. Habits

Couples, whether heterosexual or homosexual, tend to get into familiar old habits when it comes to sex – who initiates it, where it takes place, what sexual positions you use, how much you talk about it. Unfortunately (or maybe not . . .) cancer can disrupt all this.

Positions that you used to love might not work any more – whether because of pain, or a lack of confidence or body changes. You may therefore need to have a rethink – making simple, often practical changes that will free you up to enjoy sex again. These can include: keeping the light off during sex, keeping a bra on (this can prevent discomfort and/or embarrassment), using a lubricant, piles of pillows to support any weak areas, new positions, changes to the speed of intercourse (some women with issues of vaginal dryness prefer to have longer foreplay and faster intercourse).

EXAMPLES

Ways to adapt

Gary (prostate cancer survivor, 60), had problems maintaining a full erection during sex. He found that while previously he had tended to be on top during sex, that if they changed position and he lay flat during sex they both enjoyed it more.

Maria (colon cancer survivor, 34) was not in a relationship during treatment but a year after it ended she did begin a sexual relationship with an old friend. She was initially reluctant to talk about her stoma bag but with her very supportive new partner she was able to tell him that she would like to have sex but in a sideways position, where neither of them could see her stoma opening. Once they started using this position, Maria was surprised by how quickly she felt able to move on to other positions and how rapidly her sexual confidence grew.

Cancer, of course, is a challenge for both partners in a relationship. It can strain the most rock-steady couples. It can also strengthen and at times even reinvigorate a relationship. Sometimes it helps couples to see what they really value in each other.

When relationships develop major difficulties after cancer, the cancer itself is rarely the only problem. But it can be the straw that breaks the camel's back. It can be the trigger that brings more fundamental tension to the surface.

CASE STUDY

Roisin, 36, cervical cancer survivor

Radical relationship changes

Roisin, an actress, had got through cervical cancer. She recognised how amazingly supportive Lou, her partner and the father of their four-year-old daughter had been. But having recovered, Roisin spent a lot of time thinking about what she wanted from life. She realised that she loved Lou but wasn't in love with him. He was her friend. He'd been a support to her when a previous relationship broke up. Their partnership had developed almost out of convenience. Roisin realised she'd never truly been in love with Lou. Her cancer made her realise that she wanted the chance to find true love in her life. The cancer had also made her realise how strong she was. She realised she'd never really been independent – she'd always relied on a man to look after her. She felt that life was too short to spend with the wrong man. The breakup of the relationship was difficult, but both Roisin and Lou were determined to be civilised for the sake of their daughter. Roisin felt her cancer made her grow up. It made her open herself up to life, and take the leap out on her own.

If your relationship is in trouble, there are relationship and sex therapists who can help you, as a couple, to work out whether you want to save your relationship or not. They can help you to rebuild it or bring it to an amicable end. It sounds unlikely, but with the right help and support, the end of a relationship really can feel like a natural progression rather than a destructive end point.

Sex with a new partner

In real life, sex doesn't just happen in close relationships. You may have to decide whether to discuss your cancer, and how it's affected your body and sexual confidence, with someone you don't know that well at all. This can feel like a major block if you're engaged in what's supposed to be spontaneous, light hearted and fun.

It just isn't realistic to think you can always keep cancer out of the equation, even if you really are only out there for a fling with no strings attached. For a start, you may need to find explanations for any physical signs that a sexual partner might notice. Preparing some responses in advance can be very useful. You could brainstorm (in advance), all the possible explanations you could come up with, from 'I have a few battle scars', or 'I've been through the mill a bit as you can see', or 'The years take their toll', through to a clear and detailed explanation about what has happened to you and the after-effects of your cancer (see pages 169–70 for how to tell a new partner about your cancer history and its impact on your sex life).

If you don't feel able to – or don't want to – discuss your post-cancer sexual requirements, you may also have to prepare yourself for a less than ideal sexual experience. But if you have an inkling that this could turn into something more serious, then – and of course this isn't always feasible – it can help to talk to your potential partner before you become sexually intimate.

Knowing when to bring up your medical history can be tricky. You are of course much more than a cancer survivor. Cancer is a major part of who you are, but it doesn't define you, any more than your family background, relationship history or job does. There are no rules here. Nobody can tell you exactly when and how to tell a possible sexual partner about your cancer history. And nobody can give you instructions on how much detail to go into. Trusting your instinct is probably the best guide (if you can find it). But bear in mind that:

- It doesn't need to be the first thing you say about yourself.

- Everyone has emotional and physical baggage – a failed relationship, a chronic illness, a fear of commitment.

- Most people give a new relationship time to develop before they go too deeply into past history or current struggles.

Two American social workers, Page Tolbert and Penny Damaskos, who have worked with cancer survivors, describe talking about cancer with a potential new partner as 'an intimate issue – rather than a secret, or worse, a crime to be confessed' (*100 Questions and Answers about Life After Cancer: A survivor's guide*, Jones & Bartlett Publishers, 2008).

So, decide how much you want to tell, and when – in your own time. But don't leave it too late either. Your cancer history is a part of you that your potential new partner may need some time to digest. You know only too well, by now, that cancer can trigger all sorts of big emotions in other people – worry for you, worry for themselves. When a potential partner learns about your cancer they are going to have a few questions, worries and uncertainties. Be prepared for this (have realistic expectations). They are likely to be surprised, maybe a bit worried, and certainly thoughtful. If they need some time to think about what this means to them, it doesn't automatically mean they're out of the picture (don't get sucked into thinking the worst).

Talking about your cancer history and how cancer has affected your sex life is a gradual process. And it's a good idea to take it slowly. If you tell them you've had cancer then move swiftly onto a discussion of your post-cancer sexual needs, you may terrify them. Instead, you could try spreading the discussion out, perhaps like this:

- First, tell them you have had cancer and have recovered from it.

- Then, at a different time completely, tell them about any ongoing issues or problems that you've had since cancer.

- Next, perhaps on a third occasion, let them know that there are sexual issues for you.

- Finally, again at another time, have a more detailed conversation about scars, lubrication, positioning, erectile function and so on.

TIP▶

SOFTLY, SOFTLY . . . THE BENEFITS

Each step will give the other person time to digest what you're saying. It will also give you time to work out how they are taking this information. If you do manage to let them know all this before you become sexually intimate, then you are not only giving them the chance to think things through, but you are also protecting yourself. How someone responds to this says a lot about the kind of person they are. If they scarper, or seem unhelpful or unfeeling, then you are better off without them. If they handle it well, you may discover that you've found a gem.

Talking about sex and cancer with someone new requires a fine balance. The only firm rule – and yes this may seem annoyingly vague and unhelpful – is to trust your instinct whenever you can.

Overall, relationships, sex and cancer survival can be a heady mix, whether you've known the other person for five minutes or fifty years. It can all feel complicated and you'll probably worry, at times, that you're never going to find your way out, at least not together. But ultimately, if you manage to communicate about how you feel and what you need from other people, life will definitely get easier – and possibly a lot more fun.

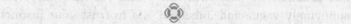

CHAPTER SIX

FATIGUE

> ❝At times, luckily not all the time, I find not only that it's hard to summon up the energy to move a muscle, but that I can't even summon up the mental energy to work out how to deal with this. It's almost as if my body and mind are both shutting down.❞
>
> **SIMON, 61, STOMACH CANCER SURVIVOR**

What is fatigue?

Fatigue isn't like any tiredness you've had in the past. It affects you both physically and mentally. It can be overwhelming, or niggling. Or it can veer between the two.

It is also the most common – not to mention the most frequently ignored – side effect of cancer and its treatment.

If you often feel:

- that sleep does not restore your energy
- weary, sapped
- like your energy suddenly drains away
- excessively tired, sometimes overwhelmingly exhausted
- unable to start or finish tasks that you want to achieve

then you are probably suffering from 'fatigue'. And it can sometimes feel uncontrollable.

If you feel this way, it's easy to imagine that you're on your own. In particular, when older cancer survivors are suffering from fatigue, other people (sometimes even including their medical teams) tend to dismiss the feeling, putting it down to age, or stress.

'People keep saying it's normal to feel like this at my age, but it's not normal for me,' says Jean, 75, colon cancer survivor. 'They say it's about time I slowed down, but they don't understand how upsetting it is for me not to be able to go to my weekly dance and exercise classes, and do the things I used to do.'

COMMON FACTS ABOUT FATIGUE

- **Fatigue is unbelievably common**. At least three-quarters of people going through cancer treatment say that they experience it, and the majority of those continue to feel fatigued after treatment ends.

- **Fatigue is hard to talk about**. Finding the words to describe fatigue can be difficult. It can feel as if no one takes it particularly seriously.

- **Fatigue is difficult to live with**. Research studies show that people find it the most difficult side effect of all.

- **Fatigue is long lasting**. Annoyingly, it is the longest lasting side effect of cancer treatment and can go on for months or even years afterwards (though – don't despair – there are many things you can do to make it feel much more manageable).

- **Fatigue is disruptive**. It can affect all areas of your life, including your physical abilities, your concentration, mood, and your relationships.

The intensity of the fatigue varies from person to person. Some cancer survivors just feel a mild dent to their energy levels, motivation and stamina. But others feel profoundly drained, unable to face even the most basic daily activities. Coming at a time when you just want your life back, this can feel like the final straw.

Why does it happen?

Fatigue is a physical and mental response to the stresses and treatments that cancer brings. It is a known side effect of certain medications used in chemotherapy. In fact, during treatment fatigue is a recognised problem and medical teams can tackle it (up to a point) with interventions including drugs and blood transfusions. But once treatment ends, and you are sent off to 'get on with your life' these interventions are usually not appropriate. So you are left feeling depleted, drained and lacking in energy, with apparently nowhere to turn.

Here are some of the long-term physical and mental effects of cancer treatment that can cause fatigue:

- **Anaesthetics and chemotherapy**: It can take a surprisingly long time to get over these.

- **Ongoing medication**: You may still be taking some medication that adds to the fatigue.

- **Your immune system or hormone levels**: These may have also changed and this, too, can cause fatigue.

- **Physical fitness**: Your body is likely to be out of condition, with weakened and under-used muscles, after cancer and its treatment. Again, this can make you feel drained and lacking in energy.

- **Sleep problems**: Disrupted sleep is very common among cancer survivors (see Chapter 7: Sleep).

- **Nutrition**: Your body has taken a huge hit, and needs to be built back up – your diet may not be giving you the energy you need. Your body may also not be using its nutrients as efficiently as it used to.

- **Low mood**: This is common after cancer (see Chapter 2: Depression and Low Mood). When you feel low you tend to lack energy or motivation.

- **Energy rollercoaster**: You could well be caught in the 'boom–bust' cycle, described below.

Emotionally drained

Cancer can also be emotionally exhausting. You have faced down a huge threat. You have been through trauma and experienced massive life changes – first in diagnosis, then during treatment. When treatment ends, you then face another massive change as you are suddenly cut loose from the support system you had become used to. Coping with all this takes vast reserves of strength, both physical and emotional. It's not surprising that you feel worn down.

Oddly, hardly anyone is actually told all this when treatment ends. Nobody really explains what fatigue is, why it's normal, and what you can do about it. Many people are left with the sense that 'it's just tiredness'. This, obviously, is upsetting – not to mention inaccurate. You think (or are told) that you should be 'bouncing back'. You're 'supposed' to get this new lease of life, do all the things you've put on hold, move mountains, reinvent yourself or, at the very least, feel like a million dollars. But you don't – in fact, most of the time, you just feel knackered.

The boom–bust trap

This is by far the most common pattern for people struggling with fatigue. Here's how it works.

You notice you have a bit more energy one day. So you get up and rush around. You do too much and exhaust yourself. The next day – or for days afterwards – you're wiped out.

It's a rollercoaster. Your life suddenly feels like it's ruled by your fluctuating energy levels. You can't build up your strength, plan or control things, because you are stuck in this boom–bust pattern. You don't know when you'll feel OK. Your body seems to have a mind of its own.

No wonder fatigue is so difficult to handle. It really can be horrendous.

CASE STUDY

Jean, 75, colon cancer survivor

Boom–bust

Jean was back at her dance class the week after her chemotherapy finished. But she was tired before the class, and wiped out after it. So, she went to bed for the next two days. On day three, when she felt she had a little more energy, she got up and embarked on the housework. Her husband had actually done it, but Jean said: 'It didn't feel right letting him do the housework. I've always done it. He does the garden and I do the house, so I wanted to show him that I was back to normal. He wouldn't have to do the housework again.'

The problem was that Jean exhausted herself again by doing the housework. She had to retire to bed for another two days. This pattern continued, much to Jean's frustration. She had fallen into the classic boom–bust trap.

How to manage fatigue

Talk to your medical team

Fatigue is an important after-effect of cancer treatment and medical teams are paying increasing attention to it. They may be able to change any ongoing medications you are on, find you nutritional advice and help you to build a safe and appropriate exercise programme (the notion of exercising your way out of fatigue may seem silly, but it isn't: see Chapter 2: Depression and Low Mood, pages 64–6, for further information).

COPING STRATEGY

The three Ps

Three Ps – Prioritise, Plan and Pace – need to become your fatigue management mantra.

1. Prioritise

This is can be a tough one. If you are a busy, independent person who likes to do things for yourself, or a 'giver' who constantly provides for other people, or a 'doer' who'll be organising and managing tons of things at any one time, then the chances are you may be struggling. Fatigue can make your life seem almost impossible. Prioritising is your first step towards picking up your juggling balls and getting them up in the air again. But to do this effectively, you may have to put some of the juggling balls to one side for a bit. It is simply not possible to pick everything back up straight away and carry on where you left off (even if you somehow managed this during treatment). So, if you work out what your priorities are, then you can make good decisions that will help you to get things moving again.

How to prioritise

Ask yourself these questions about your life and all the things you're trying to get done:

- What really needs to be done right now?

- Can anything be delayed or reduced?

- What tasks use up a lot of my physical or mental energy? Do I **need** to do these things?

- Are there people or tools that can help me? (Would a wheeled shopping bag help when I'm shopping? Can a friend carry some bags for me?)

- Which tasks are particularly meaningful for me? Which make me feel good about myself, or feel particularly personal? (For example, looking after the grandchildren or being involved in a charity?)

- Which tasks are less important or meaningful? Could I just leave these? Could someone else do them for me? (If so, who?)

TIP ▶

You'll probably need to discuss these changes with other people, explaining clearly why you're doing this. Be prepared to do some negotiating.

Watch your thoughts

Sometimes, it's not other people, but your own thoughts that stop you from managing fatigue. 'Should, must, have to' thoughts are particularly common – and disruptive (I should be able to make dinner for twelve people – I used to manage it just fine). Try to catch yourself when you're thinking these things, and question the thoughts, replacing them with kinder or more realistic ones. (See Chapter 1: Worries.)

Prioritising isn't permanent

You don't have to put things on hold or hand things over to other people forever. But while you are struggling with post-cancer fatigue, taking on too many tasks and activities will only keep you caught in the boom and bust cycle. Over time (weeks or possibly even months) you will get better at planning and pacing yourself. You'll build up your energy and strength. You'll slowly recover. And you'll find that you can take more on again.

CASE STUDY

Simon, 57, stomach cancer survivor

Prioritising

Simon is a deputy head teacher of a large secondary school. He teaches maths and IT is also responsible for exam registration, timetabling, organisation and monitoring. His wife has chronic lung disease so he has taken on many of the household tasks, including shopping and laundry. The couple are involved with their local church, hosting a weekly bible reading group and running the refreshments after the Sunday service. They have two adult children and love having their three grandchildren to stay at weekends.

Simon had surgery and chemotherapy. He was off work for six months. He made a good recovery but was left with low appetite and some eating difficulties. He also suffered from fatigue. He felt that after six months off work he should get back to school as

→

quickly as possible. And even though the school offered him a gradual return, he plunged back in full time, taking on all his previous teaching and management roles. He drove himself to and from school and did the shopping on his way home.

When he got home, he'd collapse in bed. He couldn't plan his lessons, do any of his church work or spend much time with his wife. They didn't have their grandchildren to stay any more. After four months of this Simon was at his wits' end. He felt that he was just 'existing'.

Simon and I talked a lot about prioritising. His first step in tackling his fatigue was to recognise his need to cut back. He accepted that, temporarily, he should work part-time.

He talked to the head teacher at his school and they rejigged his responsibilities, looking at which tasks he was particularly skilled at and which could be taken on by others. At home, Simon's wife began ordering groceries over the internet, and they talked to their vicar about taking on some slightly smaller jobs at church. Simon got a lift to and from school with a colleague so he wouldn't have to do the tiring drive every day. And instead of having their grandchildren for weekend visits, he and his wife decided to have them for half a day on Saturdays, just to begin with.

Simon still beat himself up about not being able to do everything he did before (he was particularly prone to 'should/ought' thinking). And he'd often end up mind reading ('I shouldn't be this tired, I should be able to pull myself out of this. Everyone's being so kind, making such adjustments for me; they must think I am a total deadweight'). We worked on this together, and he gradually learned to say kinder things to himself, for instance: 'This is only temporary. This is a step to building up again. I'm not doing

→

*what I want but I am at least doing something. Other people
don't mind helping me out – some of them are actually quite
pleased to help.' Simon accepted that there was no alternative: in
order to function better, he had to make some changes.*

*Gradually, Simon's energy levels improved, and he began to take
more on again. It was a very slow process, sometimes frustrating,
but after six months he told me, 'It's been worth it. I'm still not
100 per cent; there's still a way to go, but I feel much more in
control, much happier with life, and a lot less exhausted.'*

COPING STRATEGY CONTINUED

2. Planning

Once you've worked out (prioritised) what you need or want to
do, then you need to plan how you'll do it.

This sort of thing might sound alien to you, but you'd be
surprised at how much you already plan without realising it –
anything from setting an alarm clock to get up in time for
work, to arranging the MOT and car insurance before it runs
out. Planning a long way ahead is more common than you'd
think too – getting fit for a charity fun run; taking a course to
make yourself more employable. Really, managing fatigue by
planning isn't all that different from the things you already do.
It's just a bit more focused.

Here's how to do it

You'll need to get into the habit of making a weekly timetable.
On a Sunday, sit down and list what needs to be done in the
coming week (write this down – on a sheet of paper, your computer, your Blackberry, a calendar).

Consider the following:

- **The timescale**: What needs to be done, and when?

- **Your priorities**: What's important, what could wait?

- **The balance**: Spread activities out through each day and through the whole week so you have a balance and avoid that boom–bust overload.

- **Energy saving**: Ask yourself, are there tools or changes that will save my energy? (Can I get dressed while sitting down? Can I change my working hours to avoid the rush hour commute?)

- **Finding a companion**: It's easier to get fitter if you meet a friend for a walk; the weekly shop is easier if you have someone who can nip back to aisle one when you realise you forgot the milk. Can you find someone to do your tasks with?

- **Rewards**: Studies show that if you can make each planned step feel rewarding then you'll be more motivated with this new behaviour. A reward can be as simple as ticking off the activities on your timetable (and saying to yourself 'I did well to do that' as you tick), putting £1 into your holiday savings jar, or arranging lunch with a friend. Above all, put your rewards into your timetable. Make them part of the plan.

- **Rest time**: When are you going to rest? You have to plan this like any other activity or task. Make sure you timetable this too.

3. Pace yourself

You need to find a level of activity that is manageable for you right now – one that doesn't leave you exhausted. Working out what this level should be is easier said than done.

You might feel that your energy levels vary from hour to

hour, let alone day to day. But, the key is to balance activity with rest. You want to have a steady level of activity with regular rests each day, gradually building up your strength and stamina without going bust. To do this, it's a good idea to break up activities and goals into manageable chunks of time. You'll probably also have to question the perfectionist thoughts and expectations that push you to work too hard, do too much and go 'bust'.

Here's how to do this:

- **Put a time on it**: Think about the things you want or need to do (the things that you've prioritised). Say one of those tasks is gardening. First, work out how long you can garden for on a bad day when you feel exhausted. Have you done fifteen minutes and found it too much? If so, then maybe ten minutes of gardening is a realistic and manageable timescale to start with. Make this your baseline. You'll aim for ten minutes of gardening before a rest.

- **Limit yourself**: Do ten minutes of gardening at one time **even when you're having a good day** and feel you 'could' ('should'?) do more. Set a kitchen timer or your mobile phone alarm so you don't get engrossed and go over your time limit.

- **Alternate with rests**: Now take ten or fifteen minutes sitting down – read a gardening book or plan your sowing schedule if you want, but physically **rest**. Then do another ten minutes of gardening (set the timer again) and take a fifteen-minute tea break. Then another ten minutes of sowing your seedlings and watering (have the timer buzzing again). And **stop**. You have now achieved half an hour of gardening. It's taken you an hour overall, but if you've set the right limits, then you're not burnt out.

- **You could repeat this pattern once or twice through the day** if you want to do more gardening. Or you could do your half an hour again, the next day.

- Once you're managing this 'baseline time' comfortably (give yourself at least a week), then slowly increase the time you spend on the task itself, while keeping the rest times the same.

- Do this for each activity that you have prioritised. Each activity will have its own baseline time: gardening might be in ten-minute chunks to start with, but maybe driving or working at the computer could start at twenty or thirty minutes each, as they are less physically demanding.

- Use prioritising and planning to make it easier on yourself. Take gardening again: you could prioritise what needs to be done most urgently in your garden. Plan ahead so that you have the right tools and clothes, and you're not wasting valuable energy trying to find the rake or your hat. Are there any energy saving tools you could use, such as longer shears so you don't have to reach so high?

- Go slowly: Be prepared for some (perhaps major) frustration. But resist the temptation to go over your limits, or increase your time too quickly. If you do, you'll be back in boom–bust before you know it.

TIP ▶

IT'S NOT AS FRUSTRATING AS IT SOUNDS

This might seem like unnatural behaviour but if you think about it, you actually often pace yourself instinctively. You'll change position while sitting, or take a biscuit break when working. You're not telling yourself to do this or calling it 'rest' or setting timers for yourself, but you're doing it all the same. The plan above is simply a more radical version of what you already do without thinking.

EXAMPLE

The supermarket shop

- **Prioritise**: Do you really want or need to do this? Can you delegate it? Could you write a list for someone else? Could you order over the internet?

- **Plan**: If it is something you either have to or want to do, then you'll need to plan it. How much energy does it take? Is it one of your biggest weekly tasks, or is it, as it was for Simon, something you try to 'fit in' at the end of your day. How does it fit into your timetable: Is it a big single shopping trip? Would mid-week when the supermarkets are less crowded make sense? Or could you change how you shop and do smaller trips more often to your local shops? Also plan how you'll get there – is there a way of making the travel easier (Can someone give you a lift?). When in the shop, can you do anything to save energy? Some ideas: get a high trolley rather than a basket or one that is too deep and makes you bend and reach; make a list that corresponds with the aisles so you don't have to keep retracing your steps; get help with packing the bags at the checkout. Small things do make a difference.

- **Pace yourself**: Think about ways to break up the activity with rests. Some ideas: go to the café for a cup of tea half-way through; take a trip to the toilet for a few moments sitting down; sit for a few minutes on the seat by the pharmacy, if there is one; also, plan your rest at home afterwards – you might be able to leave the shopping in bags for half an hour while you sit down, or get someone to help you unpack.

- **Reward yourself**: Maybe you could put a treat in the trolley that will remind you that you successfully prioritised, planned and paced this shopping trip.

OK, so this all probably looks long-winded. But remember: it is the small things that together make a vast difference to your fatigue levels.

TIP ▶

PERSIST

OK, so in the real world, you might fail to plan your week on Sunday evening – and, even if you do it, unexpected things might happen – the alarm doesn't go off, a colleague is sick, your child gets sent home from school, the car breaks down. Plans aren't perfect, and you'll be in trouble if you expect to follow them perfectly. But planning can help you to regain a sense of control, particularly over the energy you use. This is why there is actually a fourth P: **Persist**. If something happens and your plan goes out the window, you might need to adjust, and have a rethink. But then you can sit back down and make a new plan. Keep going. It really works.

CASE STUDY

Jean, 75, colon cancer survivor

Jean's plan

Jean worked out that even on a day where she was feeling really drained she could manage ten minutes of housework without feeling totally exhausted. So, instead of vacuuming the whole house, as she had done shortly after finishing chemotherapy, she divided up the housework into batches of ten minutes.

➡

Initially on a bad day Jean felt that she could probably manage ten minutes every three hours. But even so, by the end of the day she'd actually achieved forty minutes of housework. She alternated between vacuuming and dusting, and even after a bad day she'd done twenty minutes of vacuuming and twenty minutes of dusting. Her house was basically clean (very clean compared to many . . .). She stuck to this time limit, even on days when she felt more energetic. This was frustrating at first, but by setting herself these daily limits she was building up her stamina. No boom–bust.

By the time we stopped meeting, Jean had built up to housework in batches of thirty minutes. She said: 'I can get plenty done and I feel like I deserve my tea break after each half hour. I think much more about what really needs to get done each day. I limit myself to three half hours of housework every day, even when I have the energy for more. I now have more time to do all the other things I enjoy, too.'

Rest and why it's vital

It's tough to even think about this. And many people struggle with the whole idea of rest. Maybe it sounds wimpy or pathetic to you. Maybe you want to keep busy: to distract yourself, to 'make the most of life'. People often worry that they might become lazy, or get bored if they just sit around resting. Perhaps you also have this burning sense that your life has been put on hold for long enough: you have to make up for lost time. Rest, then, isn't necessarily an easy idea.

As Simon (stomach cancer survivor) put it: 'Telling myself to rest just feels wrong. I've always been such an active person, rest is an indulgence. It's not something I feel comfortable with at all.' But as you've seen above, rest is a vital part of tackling fatigue.

Ways to rest without going mad:

- Call it something else if you don't like the word 'rest' ('muscle recovery time', 'taking a break', 'catch up time', 'quiet time', 'wind down time').

- See rest as one part of the whole. Yes you are having to rest, but you also have to exercise as well (see pages 194–5). Athletes build rest into their schedules and know it is as valuable as the exercise time.

- Don't confuse sleep and rest. You may wish to nap during the day but make any naps very brief, certainly never longer than twenty minutes or half an hour, especially if you struggle with sleep at night. Remember, you don't have to rest in bed and you don't have to stop everything and stare at a blank wall. You can read the paper, stretch, have a cup of tea, do a crossword or have a quick chat: these are all 'restful' things. Just think of this as an interval where you do less physically strenuous things, to balance the activity.

- Limit your rest times. Be as strict about your rest periods as you are about your activities. Set an alarm for fifteen or thirty minutes (or whatever time period you are using) when you start the rest time. Then make sure you get up and do things when the alarm goes off.

TIP▶

YOUR CONTROLLED REST PRESCRIPTION

Fatigue is not something you can push yourself out of, or force your way through. Controlled rest is a vital part of managing fatigue. Think of this page of this book as your prescription for 'controlled rest'. It's a bit like a prescription you'd get from the doctor, telling you what times of day to take your medicine and what dosage. Rest may not come out of a bottle but it helps to take your doses as seriously, and regularly, as if it did.

How to manage fatigued thoughts

The chances are you have a lot of unhelpful thoughts buzzing round your head about what you should be able to do now cancer treatment is over, or how you're failing to do the things you ought to be doing. These thoughts can make you push yourself to do too much. And, once again, this keeps you in that dreaded boom–bust cycle.

Fatigued thoughts tend to fall into familiar patterns, or 'thought traps'. (See Chapter 1: Worries, pages 17–19 for a full explanation of thought traps.)

Here are the most common fatigue thought traps:

- **High/unrealistic expectations**: 'I used to be able to do so much'; 'I should be able to do that for goodness' sake'; 'It's been X months . . . I should be over this'.

- **Self-criticism**: 'I'm hopeless'; 'I'm just making a fuss'; 'I should be able to do more'.

- **'All or nothing' thinking**: 'It is no good starting that if I can't finish it'; 'If I can't make it to work every day, my career is over'.

- **Mind reading**: 'They all think I am just being lazy'; 'Everyone thinks I'm a whinger'.

- **Fortune telling**: 'I'll never be able to do that much again'; 'I'll always feel like this'.

It's vital to identify what thoughts are making you push yourself too far. It's also important to recognise your own despairing, draining thoughts: the ones that make you wonder if you'll always be fatigued like this, if 'this is it' from now on.

The hard thing about fatigue is that no one – doctor, psychologist, friend, fellow survivor – can tell you how long it's going to last. But generally the fatigue does fade with time and if you follow this advice then you are sure to speed up that process or at least find ways to manage it, and stop it from disrupting your life.

Thought catching

Other chapters (See Chapter 1: Worries and Chapter 2: Depression and Low Mood in particular) explain in more detail how to manage your unhelpful thoughts. But when it comes to fatigue, there are a few key things to watch out for.

When you:

- find yourself feeling particularly tired and having to stop an activity earlier than you would like

- struggle to start an activity or motivate yourself to get going

- push yourself 'beyond your limits' when you know you should stop

then your thoughts are probably being particularly unhelpful – and now is a brilliant time to 'catch them' in the act.

To catch your thoughts, try to notice exactly what you are saying to yourself when the things listed above happen.

- Try to get hold of the exact words going through your mind. This isn't easy at the best of times, let alone when you're exhausted. But they are there and you can find them if you force yourself to look hard.

- Once you have 'caught' the thought, if possible write it down (this gives you a distance from it, and helps you to be more objective: on paper, it's somehow not so much a part of you as it is when it's just in your head).

- Look back at the thought traps listed above: are you falling into one?

Ask yourself these questions about that thought:

- Am I taking my circumstances into account or am I expecting to be my old, pre-cancer achieving self?
- Am I calling myself names and criticising myself?
- Is this helpful, or does it just make me feel demoralised?
- What would I say to a close friend in this situation – and why, then, am I saying something different to myself?

TIP▶

WHEN YOU REALLY HAVEN'T GOT THE ENERGY

Writing down your answers to these questions will really help, but if you haven't got the energy, just try this: Whenever you catch a thought ask yourself 'Is this fair?' 'Is this helpful?' This can help you to break out of the boom–bust cycle, giving you just a moment to challenge those awful thought traps.

CASE STUDY

Fiona, 50, leukaemia survivor

Fiona was finding it very difficult to get her life back on track. Before the cancer she was a single mother working part time in a supermarket, doing all the housework, looking after her three teenage children including one with learning difficulties. Everyone kept telling her that she was doing too much, but →

she pressed on. The cancer stopped all of this. Fiona had a very difficult time during treatment. When she came to me she had made a fair physical recovery but was exhausted. She felt that she was not managing to do anything well, and just couldn't get going again.

First of all, I asked Fiona to keep an activity record (see pages 67–8). This showed she was doing far more than she realised, but it also showed that she was in the boom–bust cycle with good days when she rushed around 'catching up' and bad days watching daytime TV in a stupor. The bad days outnumbered the good days. Fiona found it hard to prioritise, plan or pace herself because she was constantly saying to herself things like: 'This is no good; I can't even manage a twenty-minute walk, and I used to be able to manage the house, a job and three children.'

Fiona had taken no account of what she'd been through for the past eighteen months. She saw fatigue as a failure rather than the most common long-lasting side effect of cancer treatment. Her expectations were therefore harsh and unrealistic. She didn't really believe she'd ever feel better and saw asking for help as a sign of weakness, and a terrible burden on everyone else.

The first step was for Fiona to recognise exactly what she was saying to herself. Whenever she noticed her energy levels dropping she wrote down the words and phrases that were in her head. She hated doing this, but it worked: seeing it in black and white on paper made her realise just how critical she was being of herself – and how unfair. She stopped labelling herself and started acknowledging that she needed time to rebuild her strength. She found a particular phrase helpful: 'Small steps, big goals'. She also found it useful to ask herself what she'd say to

→

someone else in her situation. And she had some surprises: 'Asking my teenage children to do the washing up after dinner and to do their own laundry wasn't met with as much resistance as I expected,' she told me. 'In fact they kind of liked knowing that they were helping me.'

Fiona also had to negotiate her return to work. She wanted to go back, but was scared she might push herself too hard and fall back into the boom–bust cycle. As a cancer survivor, Fiona's employment rights were covered by the Disability Discrimination Act. Her employer therefore had to make reasonable adjustments to help her return to work (this can include adjusting work hours, exploring options to work from home, altering work tasks, gradually building up work hours, helping with travel to work options, time off for follow-up appointments etc.).

As Fiona works for a large company she had a meeting with her occupational health adviser who helped her to negotiate her return to work requirements. She went back two days a week for half a day each time, building up over three months to her previous level of three and a half days a week. She was not to do any lifting or handling work but instead varied between working on the till, supervising new employees and telephone support.

Sometimes, Fiona still finds herself thinking that her colleagues have 'forgotten all about what I have been through, and are expecting me to be back to normal'. But she'll now 'catch' this – and thoughts like it – and recognise that she is mind reading. She'll then think about what she'd say to a friend in this situation. 'It's helped me to be less prickly, and to get back into the work friendships again,' she told me. 'I feel more confident, and I'm managing my fatigue – it's much more manageable than I ever thought it could be.'

Get moving

Asking you to get some exercise may sound odd in a chapter about fatigue – surely you should be resting, not doing aerobics? But exercise is very important when it comes to tackling fatigue. Your body has been through the mill – your muscles are likely to be weaker, you are almost certainly less fit. Rebuilding your muscle strength with gradual and paced exercise will give you more, not less energy, whatever age or stage you are at. You may have huge physical challenges to overcome because of cancer treatment. It is always a good idea to talk to your medical team or GP about anything that could affect your return to fitness – this way you can fully understand any limitations or issues before you start.

Lyn, age 44, breast cancer survivor, took up running to regain fitness after cancer treatment, but she found that she struggled to improve her fitness levels. She grew increasingly frustrated – even her husband accused her of being weedy – and eventually she went to the doctor. The GP told her that radiotherapy might have damaged her lungs and that this would explain why she was struggling to see an improvement in her fitness. 'It would have been nice to know, when I was getting nowhere with my training, that my poor lung capacity was probably due to the radiotherapy,' she says. 'If someone had told me earlier, I might have revised my expectations.'

There are, however, always things you can do that will help your body to tackle the fatigue. Here's how to get moving:

- **Aim low to begin with**. Follow the rules about pacing your activities and balancing them with rest.

- **Build up very gradually**. If you've been very inactive, you can even start with just moving from sitting to standing a few times, stretching gently or taking a stroll around the block.

- **Do something you like**. You don't have to start aerobics classes – walking the dog, swimming or gardening all count as activity. (See Chapter 2: Depression and Low Mood, pages 65–6 for more information and tips about starting some exercise.)

- **Keep hydrated by drinking water during exercise**.

- **Aim to build up to about thirty minutes** of moderate activity most days of the week. Recognise that this could take time.

- **Find an 'exercise buddy'**. For instance, getting a friend to join you on your walks or whatever exercise you do can really help keep you motivated.

- **Get advice from your medical team** or get a professional consultation with a physio or sports therapist at your local sports centre. It's best to have a structure for how to build up your fitness, safely and well, without over-stretching yourself, and if you have specific physical issues to overcome, it is always a good idea to get medical advice.

TIP ▶

IT REALLY WORKS

Numerous scientific studies show that light to moderate levels of exercise (for instance, walking programmes) several times a week will improve your levels of physical activity, your appetite, your ability to function and your quality of life during and after cancer treatment. If there is one thing to do to manage your fatigue, make it exercise, but **only** if it's prioritised, planned and paced. If it isn't, you'll quickly go boom–bust.

COPING STRATEGY

Talking about fatigue

It can be very hard to talk to other people, even those close to you, about fatigue – you might worry that it sounds woolly when you try to describe it and you may be reluctant to sound like you're complaining.

1. **Be patient**. Remember that while fatigue is hard to explain it's also hard to understand. Keep going: it may take a while to convey exactly what fatigue is, and how you plan to tackle it.

2. **Convey the medical angle**. Explain that fatigue is not the same as being tired. Explain that it's recognised by doctors as a consequence of cancer and its treatments. It isn't down to a lack of sleep (or ageing) and it can't be sorted out by 'catching up on sleep'.

3. **Negotiate**. To manage fatigue, you're probably going to have to negotiate with people around you – your partner, children, friends, manager and colleagues. Two of the Ps – Prioritise and Plan – are important skills here. Prioritise what's important to you, and what you really want help with (you are going to come up against obstacles if you ask for help with everything, unless you have a local saint, and even if you do, that saint will probably irritate you after a while ...). Next, plan what you are going to ask for, and how it will work.

4. **Be clear**. Explain that fatigue is seriously affecting your life right now, but you have a clear idea about how to manage it (though this won't necessarily make it go away). Explain that the things you're asking them to do are part of a structured plan for managing your fatigue. If you give clear, specific instructions or requests ('Can you come over at 11a.m. on Thursdays and unpack my supermarket shop?'), you'll get a much better response than if you start waffling

on about change and needing help ('I have to make changes, I'm very tired'). This can also help the people close to you not to feel demoralised – your fatigue might be hard for them to handle too. In fact, try getting the people close to you to read the whole of this chapter.

5. **Stay confident**. You have every right to talk about this. And other people are probably desperate to help you anyway (it can be very hard to know how to support someone with cancer and even harder after cancer). At work, people might not feel quite so willing to pitch in (although often managers or colleagues do want to do something – they just don't know how). It can therefore be useful to prepare yourself with information about your rights and their responsibilities under the Disability Discrimination Act. The conversation doesn't have to be formal, but having solid information up your sleeve can be a useful Plan B if no one seems to be listening.

6. **Be prepared to stop**. If the conversation isn't going well, stop. Don't exhaust yourself talking if the other person isn't in the right frame of mind to listen or hear what you are saying. Arrange another time to try again.

7. **Keep talking**. If you use the strategies in this chapter, you will slowly build up your strength and stamina. So, what you need from others might change. A one-off conversation probably won't be enough. It can help to set times to review your progress and look at what you need from other people now.

8. **Thank people**. You're not asking for favours; you're giving clear information about how people can support you as you tackle fatigue. But if they are willing, and it works, then remember to thank them. If you do this, they are more likely to continue helping you (it's all about rewards again!). And people would probably also like to know that they are making a difference.

CASE STUDY

Jean, 75, colon cancer survivor

Building back up

Jean had talked to her dance teacher about how she wanted to start the classes again but was frustrated that she couldn't manage a whole class. The teacher had helped other dancers back from injury – she knew it had to be gradual. She suggested Jean go along to each weekly class but only actually do the stretch and warm up exercises at the start. Once she was managing this easily, she did ten minutes of dance. She built this up gradually, over several weeks, in five-minute add-ons until she could do the whole hour-long class again.

'It meant so much to me to get back to dancing,' Jean says. 'It was a way of putting the cancer properly behind me, of showing myself and the world that despite being 75 and having had cancer I was not beaten. But I had to learn to do it gradually and not to push myself too far or too fast. It wasn't easy. Sometimes I felt despairing. But I got there.'

Alternative therapies

People often turn to alternative therapies – such as acupuncture, reflexology and aromatherapy – to try and shake off the fatigue and tap into their energy again. The scientific evidence to prove that alternative therapies work on fatigue is not clear but sometimes it isn't research that you need; it's knowing that aromatherapy helped your friend or neighbour. If you can attend your local cancer support centre or afford nice treatments there is certainly nothing wrong with a bit of TLC – some focused time with a sympathetic and gentle therapist can make you feel a whole lot better. They can also give you really valuable rest time – not to mention the 'rewards' you need. But don't expect miracles from alternative therapies. The tried and tested ways to cope with fatigue, already outlined in this chapter, may not smell as nice as a bottle of aromatherapy massage oil, but they do work.

Memory difficulties: 'Chemobrain'

Many people report that during chemotherapy they suffer memory loss or have problems concentrating. They might struggle to find the right word, follow a fast conversation or retain information. Psychologists call these symptoms 'cancer treatment-related change in cognitive function', but many people now call these troublesome symptoms 'chemobrain'.

This is a relatively new area of scientific research, but cancer specialists are increasingly recognising that chemobrain can be a significant problem for many people, both during and after treatment. They are working on medical solutions – and ideally hope to prevent chemobrain completely.

For many people, chemobrain goes away a few weeks after chemotherapy ends. But for others it lingers much longer. It can be very upsetting to feel like you're losing your memory, but chemobrain does pass – eventually. In the meantime, there are practical ways to manage these irritating and sometimes distressing effects.

Chemobrain action plan

- **Make daily 'to do' lists**: Write a list of all the tasks you need to achieve each day. This will help you to remember what you have to do, and can also be valuable evidence that you are achieving things, even when it feels like you're not (see 'activity record', pages 67–8).

- **Leave yourself messages**: On your answerphone, mobile

voicemail, computer or just on little post-it notes around the house. These are instructions to yourself of things you need to remember (for example switch off cooker/lock front door/feed dog).

- **Get organised**: Keep objects in familiar or logical places – car keys on a hook by the garage door, mobile phone charger by your landline phone, cleaning products under the sink. Be consistent.

- **Say it and see it**: If you say out loud what you need to remember, you will activate what's known as your 'auditory memory'. If you also visualise it, your 'visual memory' will kick in too. This is a kind of memory booster system. For instance, when you put your handbag down, take a moment to look at it carefully and picture where it is. Now say out loud: 'handbag on chair by front door'. Similarly, if you are making an appointment or meeting someone new, saying their name or the appointment time, date and venue out loud while you are writing it down can really help.

- **Carry a notebook** (or use a handheld device such as a Blackberry or iPhone): Get into the habit of jotting down any thoughts, names and events that you need to remember.

- **Minimise distractions when you need to concentrate**: For instance, get out of the busy, noisy living room and sit on the stairs while you are having a telephone conversation. Ask to be moved out of the open plan office into a smaller room at work (remember your rights under the Disability Discrimination Act). Turn the radio off when you are driving. This will help you to concentrate on the important tasks.

- **Keep your brain active**: Sudoku puzzles or crosswords can help to recharge your memory banks and get you back firing on all cylinders.

- **Try not to worry:** Adding anxiety into an already challenged memory system will only make things worse. Remind yourself that this is 'chemobrain': it's a clearly recognised side effect of cancer treatment; it's not an additional illness or condition to face. It will fade. How long it takes to do so varies from person to person, but hang on in there: studies show that symptoms lessen a year after chemotherapy and decrease even more two years on. In the meantime, you have the strategies to manage this.

TIP ▶

Think back to life before cancer and try to recall how often you may have forgotten things, mislaid objects, got lost, but paid it little or no attention. Memory lapses are normal; the human brain doesn't have the capacity to retain everything.

Fatigue may be really hard to cope with, but if you can make yourself do some of the things in this chapter, you will be able to manage it better, whether it's a brief inconvenience, or much more long-lived.

Family, friends and carers: How you can help with fatigue

If you remember one thing from this chapter, remember this: **There is a big difference between 'fatigue' and 'tiredness'** (re-read the start of this chapter to understand what this difference is).

Helping with fatigue: Dos and don'ts

- **Don't** put it down to laziness, lack of motivation or 'being wimpy', and don't fall into the trap of dismissing fatigue with 'Well, you're getting older after all'. Instead:

- **Do** try to remind yourself regularly that fatigue is an extremely common, medically recognised side effect of cancer treatment. Your loved one can't do what they used to do because they are suffering from a profound lack of energy. These energy levels will build up again but this can take a very long time. Your frustration is completely understandable, but you should try to keep it under control.

- **Don't** try to do everything for them. You may well have to take on more tasks than usual but it is important not to leave the person thinking that they can't do anything. If you just take over, they may lose even more confidence, and feel very low. Instead:

- **Do** talk about what they can achieve – or have achieved – rather than what they are not managing to do.

- **Don't** be tempted to cram tons of activities into a day when they seem to have more energy than usual. This will overstretch them, and can set things back. Instead:

- **Do** develop an understanding of the boom–bust cycle (pages 175–6). Talk about how your loved one might be able to gradually build stamina. Help them to set realistic goals and to work towards these gradually. (Learn about the three Ps: pages 177–86.) It will also help enormously if you understand how they can establish a 'baseline' activity level and pace their activities accordingly (see pages 182–6).

- **Don't** say 'You have to rest!' This can be infuriating – not least for you when they don't do it. Instead:

- **Do** help them to plan their daily rest times in advance. Encourage them to see that rest does not necessarily mean 'doing nothing' (though sometimes doing nothing is a

great idea). If your loved one doesn't like the word 'rest'
then use whatever word they prefer.

Five more ways to help

1. Encourage them to exercise and build up their fitness
   gradually (see page 194). Offer to join them if you can.
   Do the same with relaxation exercises.

2. Be aware that setbacks are part of the deal when
   overcoming post-cancer fatigue. However well you've
   both prioritised, planned and paced the day there are
   going to be moments when the fatigue takes over. This
   isn't a failure on anyone's part – it's the nature of fatigue.

3. To stop them becoming demoralised when this happens,
   acknowledge that it's upsetting and frustrating but focus
   on what they're still managing to do, even during the
   setback itself.

4. Remind them of their three Ps (see pages 177–86) and if
   necessary help them to plan again how they're going to
   rebuild their energy levels.

5. Encourage your loved one to believe that while all this
   is hard, and frustrating, they can – and will – get their
   energy back. And believe this yourself – it **will** happen,
   and you **can** help.

CHAPTER SEVEN

SLEEP

> ❝ It was when I lay down in bed next to my wife who was gently snoring away, that the enormity of what we'd been through really hit me. ❞

LEN, 73, PROSTATE CANCER SURVIVOR

Diagnosis, treatment and sleep

Your diagnosis may well have changed the way you sleep. Studies show that most people with cancer wake up several times a night and at least 50 per cent of them have insomnia. It's often the quiet hours when your thoughts race or spin in circles. This can feel out of control. Even if you've always been a brilliant sleeper, cancer treatment can be extraordinarily disruptive.

SLEEP PROBLEMS DURING DIAGNOSIS AND TREATMENT

- You might find it hard to sleep on a hospital bed, in a busy ward (or even a quiet single room), while waiting for, or recovering from surgery or other invasive treatments.

- The side effects of surgical and pharmaceutical treatments – pain, nausea, vomiting, urinary frequency – may keep you awake for long stretches of the night.

- Your normal routine has been changed. You might be less active physically during treatment. Maybe you're not at work any more. Just changing the times you get up or go to bed can disrupt your sleep patterns.

- Your mood can be affected. Sleep problems can trigger depression and anxiety. But it works the other way around too: depression and anxiety can trigger sleep problems.

- During the day, noise, company and activities might distract you from anxious and worrying thoughts. But a silent bedroom in the dead of night is fertile ground for them. The pressure then builds. 'I'd lie in bed awake thinking over and over again how if I did not get myself off to sleep in the next few minutes there was no way I would be able to manage the chemotherapy tomorrow,' says Sandra, 65, vulva cancer survivor.

- If you already had a tendency to sleep badly, before the cancer, all of this is likely to be even worse, after diagnosis.

Sleep problems after cancer

But why would sleep still be a problem, now that cancer is a thing of the past?

Well, sleep is a habit. Once it's disrupted it can take time to settle again. As Sandra puts it, 'Even now, when my treatment has stopped, I am doing well physically, getting back to my busy life and having fun, I'm still lying awake in bed at night. It feels like it's the one thing that the blasted cancer disrupted, which I can't get back under control.'

COMMON REASONS WHY SLEEP CAN BE A PROBLEM AFTER TREATMENT ENDS

- **Ongoing after-effects of treatment**: Some of these become particularly troublesome at night. For example, pain or discomfort from scars or weakened muscles, temperature changes, night sweats, urinary or bowel frequency. 'I get off to sleep OK but then I wake in the early hours of the morning drenched in sweat and boiling hot,' says Alice, 54, a breast cancer survivor. 'I have to stand by my window, which I open wide whatever the weather. Often the sweats are so bad I have to change my nightdress and entire bedding. By this time, I'm wide awake again. It's hell. I'm exhausted all the time, tetchy, irritable – really quite despairing at times. All because I can't get any sleep.'

- **Emotions**: There are many big emotions when treatment ends, and there's nothing like the middle of the night for making these even more intense. Worries about the cancer coming back, a low or depressed mood or racing thoughts all tend to get worse at night, and can keep you awake until the wee hours. 'I've been so strong through all of this,' says Callum, 51, kidney cancer survivor. 'That's why I find it so surprising that it's only now – when I've been given a clean bill of health – that I'll lie in bed at night worrying about all the different outcomes there might have been – or could still be.'

- **Worries about sleep itself**: It's a vicious circle, because you worry about not sleeping, and the act of worrying itself keeps you awake. You fret about what your lack of sleep will do to you – how you'll cope the next day, how long you can function without a good night's sleep. 'I lie in bed worrying about how I am going to be able to drive the forklift truck at work tomorrow morning,' Callum continues. 'I worry about whether I'll be a danger to myself and others, and whether I'll be even more of a grumpy old so and so than I usually am to my poor wife and kids. Then I know I'll never sleep, I'm so keyed up.'

For some cancer survivors sleep isn't a problem at all. It just goes back to normal. They feel rested and restored after their good nights' sleep.

They are the lucky ones.

For many, many others, good sleep can feel like a distant fantasy.

Sleep basics

Understanding the basic facts about sleep can really help you to tackle your sleep problems.

Sleep patterns

Your sleep patterns are strongly influenced by your twenty-four-hour 'body clock', also known as your 'circadian rhythms'. These rhythms have a major effect on your sleep patterns. They encourage you to sleep when it is dark and wake in the morning when the sun has risen.

Night shift workers, airline staff who fly overnight, and other people whose sleep does not fit the traditional pattern of night-time sleeping and daytime waking, can struggle to return to night-time sleeping patterns when their lifestyle changes. Their body clock has been disrupted. Their habits have changed. The same goes for cancer recovery. You've developed some new (and largely unhelpful) habits. You need to change them back.

What is 'normal sleep'?

Sleep is a basic human requirement – like water and food. You can't live without it.

Sleep is made up of a series of cycles that repeat throughout the night.

Most of us think sleep is constant – just a period of time doing nothing. But it's not really an episode of inactivity at all – far from it. There are actually lots of physical and mental processes going on during sleep.

NORMAL SLEEP PATTERNS

The normal adult sleep pattern goes like this:

1. A fairly rapid transition from being awake, to falling asleep.

2. A quick transition into deep sleep.

3. The longest and deepest part of the sleep cycle. This lasts approximately four hours. Sleep experts say that you get the biggest benefit from these early, deep sleep episodes. (This perhaps explains why Mrs Thatcher was famously able to function on only four hours of sleep a night!)

4. The rest of the sleep cycle: peaks and troughs between deep and lighter sleep episodes until you wake up.

Common sleep myths

Sometimes, we make sleeplessness worse by beating ourselves up about how much sleep we 'need' when in fact the reality is far less intimidating.

- **Myth**: If you lose sleep, you have to catch up the same amount, or you'll stay tired.

- **Fact**: Experts say you don't need to catch up on all the sleep you've lost, if you've had a bad night. Just getting an initial period of good quality deep sleep – at the start of a night – is enough.

- **Myth**: We need eight hours a night to function properly.

- **Fact**: You may actually need far less than this. Five or six hours' sleep could be perfectly fine.

- **Myth**: Daytime fatigue means I'm not getting enough sleep.

- **Fact**: For cancer survivors fatigue may have many different causes that are nothing to do with night-time sleep (see Chapter 6: Fatigue). If you find yourself exhausted during the day, it may not be down to poor sleep at night.

How much sleep do I actually need?

You may need less sleep than you think. The amount of sleep you need changes during your lifetime. Not everyone needs the same amount of sleep. So, the figures below represent average nightly sleep needs:

- adolescent – nine to ten hours
- adult – seven to eight hours
- older adult – six to seven hours.

Insomnia

Insomnia is a term used to describe any or all of the following sleep difficulties:

- difficulty falling asleep (more than half an hour after going to bed)

- frequent night-time waking (more than twice a night)
- waking early in the morning.

You might find yourself struggling to cope with a combination of the difficulties listed above. And you may also find that though you manage to get to sleep and stay asleep, you don't feel restored by sleep.

Sleep problems can be incredibly frustrating and depressing but sometimes worrying that you aren't getting enough sleep is actually more of a problem than the amount of sleep you are getting. The body is designed to handle a certain amount of sleeplessness.

Changed habits

Sleep is a habit. Changing habits can be hard. So, once your sleep patterns are disrupted – by diagnosis, treatment and then survival-related issues such as anxiety – it can be very difficult to get your old good habits back. But you can do it.

TIP ▶

FOOD, BOOZE, COFFEE AND CIGARETTES

Many people try to use food and drink to help themselves get off to sleep. This tends to backfire. When Hamish, 72, prostate cancer survivor, noticed that he felt sleepy after his big lunch and glass of beer he swapped things around, so he had his big meal and beer late in the evening. This made things worse. Large meals an hour or two before bed don't help you to sleep. If your body is struggling to digest, it won't rest. So, try to eat a light meal early in the evening so that your body has time to cope with the food. The same goes for alcohol – you may think alcohol makes you sleepy. It can, at first, but studies show that alcohol triggers night-time waking – so you are likely to find yourself awake later on in the night. So, keep your alcohol intake to a minimum: maybe just the one glass of wine with your (early) dinner.

Most people know that caffeine is a stimulant. But it's important to remember that caffeine isn't just found in coffee but also in tea, colas, chocolate and even in smaller amounts in decaffeinated coffee. You could try limiting caffeine to mornings only. Similarly, nicotine is a stimulant – smoking can keep you awake along with all its other damaging effects.

CASE STUDY

Andrea, 53, bowel cancer survivor

Racing thoughts

Andrea is an immigration officer who completed her bowel cancer treatment six months before being referred to me by her clinical nurse specialist.

She told me that she felt more exhausted now than she had done at any point in her treatment. She was managing to work but she knew that the quality of her work was being damaged by her sleep difficulties. Her relationship with her sixteen-year-old son was suffering, too; she was more irritable with him, less enthusiastic about doing the things they used to enjoy together, such as ice skating or going to the cinema. Her husband was supportive, but his work had taken him abroad and he was rarely at home.

→

It would take Andrea one to two hours to drop off to sleep. She'd then wake several times in the night, feeling tense and wound up. In the morning, she did not feel refreshed at all.

She knew that her worrying was making it difficult for her to fall asleep. 'When I get into bed at the end of a long day I become much more aware of my body and any twinges or gurgles it makes,' she said. 'I do know it's probably my muscles unwinding after a long stressful day, and that I'm paying more attention to my gut than I do during the day when I'm busy and able to distract myself. But I can't help it; I just start to worry about what's happening inside me.'

She also worried about the sleep difficulties themselves. 'My head hits the pillow and I immediately start to wonder how long I'll be lying like this for. I then look back over my day, remembering how tired I felt and wondering if I made mistakes at work because of this. Then I remember how I snapped at my son and I feel guilty. I think if only I could get a couple of good nights' sleep all this would seem so much better.'

Andrea's experience is incredibly common. Together we identified the various causes of her sleep problems, and worked on strategies to overcome them. Andrea found the sleep diary (page 213) a great starting point – it helped her to understand her own habits more clearly. She also realised how important 'wind down time' was (page 215) and started to build that into her evening, along with some regular daily exercise (she started walking the twenty minutes to work instead of taking the bus). These strategies are all outlined in this chapter. It wasn't always easy, but six months on, Andrea no longer has problems sleeping. She feels, she says, 'like a completely different person: stronger, more reasonable, more able to cope.'

How to tackle your sleep problems

The first step in tackling any sleep problem is to understand it. To do this, it is a good idea to keep a record of your sleep patterns. This way, you can start to 'unpick' what's going on for you.

Sleep is very hard to actually monitor for yourself (time creeps when you're lying awake at night). It can also be hard to know if your sleep is improving, without any objective proof. This is why the first step to tackling your sleep problems is to keep a sleep diary.

COPING STRATEGY

Your sleep diary

Keep a notepad by your bed. Each night, jot down:

* what you are doing for the couple of hours before you go to bed

* what time you go to bed

* what time you turn the light off

* what time you go to sleep*

* the number of times you wake in the night

* what time you wake up and get out of bed to start the day

* any daytime naps you had, either planned or unplanned.

*Clearly, what time you go to sleep is going to be an estimate, made the following morning – the last thing you need after finally dropping off is to wake up to note what time you went to sleep!

Also use your sleep diary to note:

- specific thoughts that are keeping you awake

- upsetting dreams

- thoughts or instructions that pop into your head about what you need to do the next day.

Why bother?

Your sleep diary will help you to identify behaviour and thoughts and understand how they are affecting your ability to sleep at night. This will help you to sort out some of the root causes of your sleep problems.

'I had never noticed before I kept my sleep diary that I spend so much time in my bed when not trying to sleep,' says Andrea. 'I've got into the habit of reading in bed so I'm not disturbed by my son watching TV in the living room. This means I spend a long time in bed before I'm even sleepy. I also speak to my husband on the phone each night when I'm in bed. Again, I realised this is something that keeps me feeling quite wakeful.'

Releasing body tension

Sleep problems can make you incredibly tense, physically. This, in turn, directly affects your ability to go to sleep, and to stay asleep. You toss and turn, twitch and thrash – you get more and more tense and jittery. It is anything but restful.

One major key to good sleep is to find ways to relax your body and to release all that tension. Some of this can be done just before bed, some while you are in bed and some during the day when you aren't even thinking about bed.

COPING STRATEGY

Step 1

Before bed: Wind down time

Establishing a 'wind down time' for the last hour or so before bed is vital. You undoubtedly already know what activities wind you up (Catching up on work? Tidying the kitchen?), so make it your straightforward rule to avoid these during that hour. This may sound simple, but it can actually be surprisingly hard to achieve. You really have to think about it, and change your habits.

In the hour before bed avoid 'wind up' activities such as:

- work

- starting potentially awkward conversations

- answering the phone

- playing a competitive or violent computer game

- watching a scary DVD or TV show.

Instead, think about what helps you to wind down physically.

Wind down ideas

- Watch a light DVD or TV programme.

- Listen to soothing music.

- Have a warm bath.

- Flip through a magazine.

- Make a warm, milky drink.

- Use a foot spa/back massage cushion.

- Any combination of the above, or anything else that you know winds you down.

CASE STUDY

Andrea, 53, bowel cancer survivor, part 2

Sleep diary

Andrea's sleep diary helped her to see that she did not really have a clear wind down time for the hour or so before bed. If anything, she increased her activity before bed, clearing up the dinner she and her son ate earlier, checking her bag and diary for the following day (which would then remind her of the coming pressures). Then there would be her call with her husband. While Andrea loved talking to her husband, it made her sad because they were apart. It also triggered quite a lot of mental activity as they'd have to discuss difficult family, work or financial situations during these calls.

In our sessions together, Andrea worked out how to change her evening pattern quite significantly. She developed a really effective wind down routine. The hour before bed was her time to cuddle her son on the sofa while listening to music (something they both really enjoyed). She'd then have a hot bath with oils recommended by an aromatherapist. She spoke to her husband on the phone shortly after she came in from work and then sent a loving text message to him before bed. She cleared dinner immediately after she and her son had eaten and organised her work bag before cooking dinner.

Andrea noticed her sleep patterns change. She began to fall asleep without such effort and, mostly, she stayed asleep all night. As a result she felt much more rested, and able to cope. 'The changes haven't just improved my sleep,' Andrea told me. 'They've made the whole atmosphere of my evenings so much better, and my days are more manageable now I'm not exhausted all the time.'

COPING STRATEGY

Step 2

During the day: Regular exercise

Taking regular exercise during the day can also do wonders for your night-times:

- Exercising during the day releases physical tension. It uses up energy so that you are not only physically tired but also more relaxed when bedtime arrives.

- Exercise can improve your mood – when you exercise, your body releases endorphins or 'feel good' chemicals. This can make you feel happier and less stressed. In fact, studies show that exercise can be just as effective as medication for mild to moderate depression.

- Exercise can also make you feel like you've achieved something during the day. This can be a big bonus if you can't stop thinking you aren't achieving enough, or are somehow 'failing'.

When should I exercise?

Exercising strenuously too close to bedtime is a really bad idea. It can 'pump you up' or energise you, and get in the way of good sleep. The afternoon or, at the latest, the early evening, are the best times to exercise in order to boost your chances of a good night's rest.

How much should I exercise?

It's important to learn, gently, what your body can handle post-cancer. If you do too much too soon you can set yourself up for some very stressful symptoms – aches and pains and even injuries. None of this is going to help you to sleep better.

Ideally, you want to rebuild your strength and energy levels gradually – so start any form of exercise slowly (you might also want to get advice from your doctor). See Chapter 6: Fatigue (page 194) for more on this.

In general, depending on your physical abilities, personality and situation, it is best to aim for about twenty to thirty minutes of 'moderate intensity' activity on most days of the week. Brisk walking or swimming are great forms of exercise. But it does not have to be anything particularly organised or formal. For the maximum benefit, you just want to be warm and slightly out of breath (not gasping: you should still be able to have a conversation). It is fine to break up your activity into two or three ten-minute slots if that's easier. Vigorous housework or gardening will do just as well, as will getting off the bus a few stops early, or energetically washing the car.

COPING STRATEGY

Step 3

In bed: Relaxation strategies

Once you actually get into bed, there are lots of good ways to relax so that you fall asleep more easily.

These can take practice, but they really do work. The best thing about using these strategies in bed – as opposed to using them for stress relief or coping with nerves and anxiety during the day – is that this time you actually **want** to fall into a deep and lasting sleep.

For a full run down of relaxation strategies see Chapter 8: Relax.

Good relaxation techniques for sleep

All of the techniques in Chapter 8: Relax are useful for sleep problems, but when it comes to sleep, start with 'muscle squeeze–release' (pages 238–42), possibly coupled with 'visualisation' (pages 243–7). Doing 'muscle squeeze–release' in bed in a darkened room, and using it to fall fast asleep is really luxurious (mostly, with relaxation exercises, you need to stay awake afterwards, in order to get on with your day). If you aren't asleep at the end of muscle squeeze–release, add the 'visualisation' technique. Most people find that if they are not fast asleep at the end of this they are well on their way to dropping off. If you're currently struggling to fall asleep this is going to be a welcome contrast to what's happening now.

TIP ▶

DON'T WORRY ABOUT TECHNIQUE

Some people worry that they aren't doing the muscle squeeze–release technique 'the right way'. **There is no right way**. Every psychologist or relaxation therapist has their own way of teaching these exercises. Every person who learns them will adapt them to suit their own needs. Turn to pages 238–40 for instructions on how to do these techniques, but don't get obsessed with 'doing it right'.

Sleep associations: What *is* your bed for?

Good sleepers associate their bed with sleep. Poor sleepers generally associate bed with all sorts of other activities – watching TV, working, eating, drinking, sex, lying awake worrying.

For cancer survivors these bed associations can be particularly tricky, not to mention harmful when it comes to sleep. You may have come to associate your bed with illness – there might be unpleasant memories such as nausea, vomiting, pain or fear.

Bed might have become a place where you worry and fret, feel lonely and scared. None of this exactly promotes a restful night.

The key to changing this is simple. You need to retrain your body so that you **associate bed with sleep**. How? Well, it's straightforward: you have to spend less time in bed awake.

Get off the bed!

Your bed should be used for two things and only two things – sleep and sex (yes, sex encourages sleep afterwards, so it's one activity that **is** allowed in bed).

Your sleep diary will have helped you to identify how you currently use your bed. You may have discovered that you sit on your bed, or lie in it – doing things other than sleeping – much more than you imagined.

Many of us see the bedroom as a quiet haven in a noisy family home. We sneak up to bed to read a book or work or think or escape. Bed then becomes associated with these activities.

A cup of tea or breakfast in bed can be an amazing gift – wonderful if you are a good sleeper or as an occasional treat. But if you are a poor sleeper and you regularly eat and drink in bed, then hey presto!, you are going to associate bed with digestion – not sleep.

Similarly, if you have a TV in your bedroom and watch it lying in bed, if you read in bed before turning off the light, or catch up on paperwork, or talk on the phone then the advice is simple: don't.

You don't need to withdraw from your bedroom completely. Just get off the bed itself.

TIP ▶

THE CALM CHAIR

Rather than rearranging your TV, bookshelves or private quiet time, see if you can possibly make yourself almost as comfy by putting a chair – or even sofa if you have space – next to your bed. You then sit wrapped up warm and cosy in a dressing gown or blanket to watch the TV, read your book or have a quiet chat.

Only get into the bed itself when you feel ready to sleep.

CASE STUDY

Hazima, 39, bladder cancer survivor

Only use your bed for one (or – OK – two) things

Hazima had terrible trouble falling asleep. Sometimes she would lie awake worrying, until 3 or 4a.m. She told me she couldn't cope during the day, with her two young children; she was strung out and exhausted.

We identified, using the sleep diary, that Hazima used her bed for a whole range of things, other than sleep, including reading, working, making calls or catching up on household admin.

Hazima had a big bed in a small room. She felt it was her only place to escape from the kids, TV, dog, noise and domestic demands. She said there was not enough space in the room for a comfy armchair, but came up with the idea of borrowing her daughter's big bean bag. She leant it against the side of the bed and found that it was surprisingly comfortable. She'd snuggle up and read on it when the kids were with her husband, or in bed. This change, along with establishing wind down time (no tasks!) helped her to relearn how to fall asleep.

→

> *It is worth noting here that some psychologists recommend not using your bedroom for anything except sleep (and sex), but in my experience, I have found that most people don't need to keep out of their bedrooms until they go to bed. Indeed, for many people, like Hazima, their bedroom is a cosy and relaxing place – maybe the only place where they can wind down in the midst of a hectic family home.*

Don't lie there and fester!

This may sound easier said than done. But, again, the basic idea is that you do not want to associate bed with worry, or with lying awake. So, you need to limit the time you spend in bed awake.

Sleep problems bring vast numbers of worries with them – starting from 'Will I get off to sleep OK tonight?' and moving through a downward spiral to 'I will never be able to sleep, my day tomorrow will be ruined: this is a total nightmare'.

Add to this your many possible cancer-related worries, and it is not surprising that you can find yourself lying in bed at night wide awake and worrying. In fact, you can quickly get so fraught that the mere process of putting your head on the pillow triggers anxious thoughts.

The key, here, is to get out of bed after fifteen to twenty minutes of sleeplessness.

In the short term this can be painful. But in the long term it really is worth it.

Hauling yourself out of the warm cosy place where you could stay comfortably – if only you were able to get to sleep – might feel like the wrong thing to do. But it is very important to get out of bed if you're not sleeping.

Do not be tempted to spring up and start doing all the tasks you didn't manage today or 'frontloading' for tomorrow. Far from it. When you are out of bed, you should be aiming for an exaggerated version of 'wind down time':

- **Find somewhere warm** – the beanbag, cushion or armchair – and just sit quietly, with dim lights, until you feel ready to try to get back into bed. This is your ideal.

- **Try something gentle**: If just sitting quietly is unhelpful, it's fine to flick through a magazine, listen to some music (headphones are handy here) or do some relaxation exercises.

- **Be prepared**: If you have night sweats or feel overheated, put something next to your 'cosy chair' that helps cool you down – iced water, some wet wipes or a mini fan. You could also have a bigger fan on through the night, and make sure there's good, cool ventilation in the room. If you know you may have to change your night clothes or bedding during the night, keep some clean replacements by the bed so you don't have to rifle through cupboards at 3a.m. Alice, 54, a breast cancer survivor, had to change her pyjamas and bedding most nights. This involved waking her poor partner as well. Alice worked out what level of dampness was bearable for her. She decided that on some occasions changing her pyjamas was enough – she didn't have to do the whole bed. She worked out that she could use two single sheets on the double bed, and when she did need to change the bed, she kept sheets right next to the bed, so everything took less effort.

TIP ▶

> Try not to fall asleep when you are out of bed! You don't want to start thinking of that cosy chair, sofa or beanbag as a sleep place. When you start to feel sleepy, get back into bed and repeat the process.

COPING STRATEGY

Worries and sleep

Your mind quickly gets involved in sleep problems. Worries spiral, and these make the problems worse. Apart from worrying about the effects of not sleeping, people often find that at night, cancer-related worries, as well as other stresses, really kick in. If this is happening to you, then what you need is a way to get your mind under control, and stop it from sabotaging your sleep patterns.

Step 1: Thoughts are not facts

The first thing to do is to remind yourself that thinking something will not make it happen (see Chapter 1: Worries, page 17). Also remember that thoughts are not facts. Instead of going with your spiralling thoughts, try to remind yourself of the sleep facts below.

Key sleep facts

Sleep studies show that:

- you do not need to catch up on all lost sleep

- we can function perfectly well with less sleep than we'd think

- it is normal for sleep to be interrupted once or twice a night

- we have our deepest and most restorative sleep in the first two to four hours of the sleep cycle.

Step 2: Thought management (the pink elephants again)

You already know that if you tell yourself not to think something, it usually has the opposite effect – remember those pink elephants on pages 29–30? So, telling yourself not to worry or think certain things at night really isn't going to work.

Instead, try the following tactics.

(i) Thinking time

If you know the thoughts that trouble you at night, try giving yourself some thinking time (maximum twenty minutes) just before you start your wind down routine. If, for instance, you notice that you tend to think about the day you've just had, and then fret about the day ahead, try writing a brief review of your day. Then outline a plan for the next day. This way, when the thoughts crowd into your head at night, you don't have to push them away or ignore them (fat chance). You can greet them calmly – tell yourself you've already thought about them. You don't need to go over it again now.

'This was a great strategy for me,' says Callum, 51, kidney cancer survivor.'I used to find myself reviewing the old day and writing lists in my head for the following day. I found that if I'd already written those lists down it was as if it settled my mind. I felt more confident that I would not forget those lists – and that confidence allowed me to slow my mind down enough to sleep.'

(ii) Write down that pesky thought

It can be extremely helpful to write persistent thoughts down, when they trouble you at night. You will already have a notebook by your bed for keeping your sleep diary notes (see pages 213–14). Just use it to write down the thoughts that keep bothering you. Sometimes intrusive thoughts become repetitive. This is because your brain wants to hang on to that thought in some way. You are worrying that sleep is going to make you forget that thought. But if your brain knows that this thought is written down, it seems to be able to turn off its repeat button. The intrusive thought is put away for the night.

(iii) Tell yourself not to go to sleep

Although this sounds counter-intuitive, it really works for some people. It's the opposite of pressurising yourself to get off to sleep. It's worth a try anyway.

Step 3: Changing your sleep habits

Daytime napping

There is strong research evidence that short naps during the day (ten to twenty minutes maximum) can re-energise your mind, without disrupting night-time sleep. However, 'short' is the key word here. If you nap for more than a maximum of twenty minutes, this will make it harder to sleep at night, which is the last thing you want.

If you feel you need a daytime nap, set an alarm for fifteen to twenty minutes, or get someone reliable to wake you (they do have to be reliable though!). Don't give in to the temptation to sleep just a 'few minutes' longer. If you find that you can't keep nap times to twenty minutes or less, it is better to ban them entirely.

Fixed bedtime

People often think that if it's hard to go to sleep, you should stay up later so you're really tired. This is a sensible strategy for those odd occasions when sleep eludes you. But if you are regularly struggling to get to sleep, if sleeplessness has become a habit, then it doesn't work so well. What you actually need is a reasonable nightly bedtime.

Think back to a time when you were sleeping well (if there is one): what time were you going to bed? If there is a big difference between this time and the time you are going to bed now, try to find a midway compromise. Now, stick to this time. Don't go to bed earlier if you feel tired, and don't stay up later if you feel alert. You are trying to train your body and mind to develop good habits. Apart from anything else, a regular bedtime stops you thinking too much about how tired you are – or are not. You don't have to go through a decision-making process every night about when to go to bed.

Fixed get up time

The same goes for mornings – have a regular time for getting up, whatever has happened during the night. Again you'd think that if you haven't slept well, then a lie in is a good idea. It isn't. A lie in skews your sleep pattern. It will then be harder to get off to sleep that evening. Work out a reasonable getting up time (this may depend on what you have to do in the morning, what time you tended to wake up before cancer disrupted your sleep, what time you have been sleeping until recently, what time you go to bed and what you think your sleep needs are: see page 209).

Then stick to this – weekdays **and** weekends. Have an alarm or a reliable person (preferably one with a thick skin and strong muscles who can drag you out of bed even though you've finally got to sleep!). Again this can be painful, but it's vital if you're to build good sleep habits. Once you've cracked your sleep problems you can have the odd lie in again, but not before.

Medication ('sleeping pills')

Sleeping pills can be fine for occasional use. But they do not help you to re-establish good sleep habits and some can become addictive when you use them for more than a few weeks. You may, very appropriately, have been prescribed some sleeping pills during your cancer treatment and they might have been really helpful. But it is important to know that if you use sleeping pills over a long time this can then trigger 'rebound insomnia' – when you stop using the pills you can't sleep.

If your sleep problem is caused by pain, night sweats and other physical symptoms such as lymphoedema or nausea it's a good idea to talk to your doctor. It may be that your doctor can manage and improve these symptoms medically. But even if you manage the body symptoms it can still take a while to get back into good sleep habits. The strategies in this chapter should still be helpful though.

Knowledge is power

If you have understood the basics about sleep – you know your sleep needs, sleep facts and the myths about sleep – you are halfway there. And if you have a range of techniques to try, then you are likely to feel very differently about your sleep problems. When you find yourself lying in bed at night struggling to get off to sleep, or waking for the umpteenth time, you'll know what to do. You'll be able to stay cool, calm and collected (despite any night sweats); reassure yourself, defuse annoying thoughts, step away from the bed, regroup and try again.

'Although I didn't like the idea of getting up in the night, I was surprised to discover that it was actually very helpful,' says Meilin, 72, a uterine cancer survivor. 'I felt as if I was doing something positive to try to help my sleep instead of lying in bed just willing myself to nod off.'

The changes may be slow to come, and these techniques can feel really difficult and annoying at first. You might have to change some deeply ingrained habits, and tackle some really difficult issues – and that's never easy.

But reminding yourself that you have a plan, and you are following it, really can get you through those tough nights.

'I'm not a perfect sleeper,' says Meilin. 'I'm not what I was before cancer, when I could sleep at the drop of a hat, anywhere, any time. But I'm a whole lot better than I could be. I'm coping when I can't sleep. And most of the time I'm getting plenty. At the end of the day, that's what matters.'

Family, friends and carers: How you can help with sleep difficulties

Trying to support someone with sleep difficulties can be really hard. Sleep is a private and individual activity, and you can't control how someone else sleeps. But if the cancer survivor is your partner, then their sleep difficulties can have a major impact on your life too. The good news is that there are many things you can do to improve things – for both of you.

- **Learn the sleep facts** (page 209): Try to reassure yourself that disrupted sleep is not as damaging as it can feel, for either of you. This can help to take some of the anxiety out of your own situation.

- **Read the strategies in this chapter**: Talk to your partner about what approach they are planning, then try to support their efforts. If, for instance, you've agreed that your partner will not lie in bed awake for more than twenty minutes, then don't make a fuss if they get out of bed – or tell them to get back in.

- **Keep night-time interactions to a minimum**: Even if you're both awake at 2a.m., don't get into any significant conversation – only talk very briefly to check if they are OK, or to ask if they need any help.

- **Encourage an evening 'wind down time'** (page 215): Make it your rule to respect this. Don't disrupt, distract or otherwise interfere when it is wind down time – it's a vital part of re-establishing healthy sleep habits.

• **Be prepared to make some temporary night-time changes**: You may need to invest in ear plugs, change the bedding or room temperature, or even consider separate beds or different rooms while your partner is re-establishing good sleep habits.

Separate rooms: Five important points

If you jointly decide that the most practical thing is to sleep in different rooms for a bit then consider the following points.

1. **Make sure that you both want this**: You've been through enough already as a couple, and altering sleeping arrangements (even temporarily) can be very emotional.

2. **Be the one to move**: Your partner has to stay in the usual bed, so unfortunately you're the one who's going to have to move. This is because your partner needs to retrain his or her body and mind to sleep in that bed and bedroom. It won't be helpful to either of you in the long term if they learn to sleep on the living room sofa bed.

3. **Make time for each other during the evening**: If you usually have a chat or a cuddle last thing at night make sure that you still have this time – just have it a bit earlier and not in bed. Changing sleep arrangements can make you feel distant so it's important to keep communicating, and touching each other.

4. **Set a time limit** for how long you are going to sleep separately and stick to it (perhaps two or three weeks). Even if your partner's sleep is still disrupted, move back into bed together for two or three weeks. Then, if you both agree, try the separate beds again. It can take several

goes, but it is better to have disrupted sleep for a while, than a physically and emotionally distant relationship.

5. **Help your partner to build up their daily exercise routine**, and establish their evening relaxation plan. Both of these will have a major impact on night-time sleep. If you can then keep them company as they exercise or practise relaxation techniques – both will be incredibly helpful to you, too, if you are tired and frustrated.

CHAPTER EIGHT

RELAX

> ⁶ My hot flushes were debilitating in so many ways; a real source of misery. But I learnt a simple visualisation technique for managing them and now I feel I'm in control again. It did take practice and didn't come easy at first, but now it's second nature to me. I still get the hot flushes but they just don't bother me like they did. I know I can deal with them. ⁷
>
> **LINDA, 60, BREAST CANCER SURVIVOR**

Relax, dammit!

'Just try to relax.' Ah, those four little words. It's hard to think of anything that is more likely to produce instant tension.

People have, no doubt, said 'relax' to you many times during your cancer treatment – usually when you're facing some unpleasant procedure or other. It is pointless to be told 'try to relax' when your fight or flight response has already kicked in. In fact, these words are pretty much guaranteed to send your stress levels skyrocketing even further.

If there was a ban on 'just try to relax', many unpleasant procedures would go far more smoothly. Instead, health professionals could be taught to say this far less snappy but far more useful sentence:

> Try to breathe in through your nose for a count of 4, hold your breath for 3 and breathe out through your mouth for 6 or 7.

This gives you a concrete strategy – something to focus on. It gives you a practical, simple way to manage the tension that's shooting through your body and mind.

What we all need, when dealing with fear, anxiety, anger, stress or indeed any of the difficult emotions discussed in this book, are simple strategies that defuse tension and generate calm. 'Relax, dammit!' is not one.

In short, simple, effective relaxation skills are the key to managing a whole range of difficult situations and emotions. If you can learn and practise some of the techniques in this chapter you will find it so much easier to get your life back on track. They are a vital part of any cancer survivor's toolkit.

How to unwind

You may be thinking 'but I already know how to wind down; I have my own way of doing this'. That's great. No one is going to try to stop you doing what works for you.

Common wind down methods you might already use include:

- having a long, hot bath
- taking a stroll round the park
- reading a book or magazine
- listening to soothing music
- spending some time in prayer

- aromatherapy
- a massage
- a meditation session
- a game of football
- a glass of wine or cup of cocoa
- listening to those whale music CDs
- a chat with a friend.

These things are really helpful. But there is one problem: they are not always practical at the exact moment you need them most.

This is why it is important also to have a handful of simple skills that you can pull out whenever your tension levels rise.

Trying to 'just relax' without these specific techniques, especially when you're in a stressful situation, is nigh on impossible, even for the most well-balanced, chilled and sane individual.

Relaxation, in short, is a skill. You can learn it, just like you learn knitting, Sudoku or how to ride a bike. Like any skill, it takes time to develop; you have to practise. But once you've really got it, it can become second nature.

TIP ▶

KEEP GOING

Don't give up if you find it hard to develop these skills at first. Most people do find it difficult. If you're already tense (and after what you have been through, this is quite likely) then it can take longer, and be even harder. But don't give up. Persevere and you'll find that you've developed an incredibly powerful way to influence your mood, cope with difficulties and boost your well-being.

Reality check

Learning to relax is not a golden ticket to a life of Zen-like calm.

No matter how honed your relaxation skills become, you are still going to be affected by the tough stuff life throws at you. You'll still say the wrong thing sometimes, make mistakes, get tense and upset or, even, when life is really hard, distraught. The difference is that with relaxation skills you will cope better, bounce back quicker, and generally feel far more in control than you would without them.

WHAT RELAXATION SKILLS CAN DO FOR YOU

Your relaxation skills will not just help you to remain alert and focused during stressful moments, they'll also help you to cope better with life in general, because you will be able to wind down properly afterwards.

During stressful situations, good relaxation skills can help you to:

- take a moment or two to remember that, deep down, you have a way to cope with this

- keep the worst fight or flight symptoms at bay

- keep some sense of control over what's happening to you.

Afterwards, good relaxation skills will help you to:

- physically – and mentally – wind down

- achieve a much deeper form of calm

- sleep better

- communicate better

- cope better with what happened.

Your relaxation toolkit

Use this basic toolkit every day. Learn these skills, practise them and see the difference in how you cope.

Skill 1: Slowed breathing

- **Myth**: To relax you have to lie down in a darkened room and imagine you're on a desert island.

- **Reality**: Lying in a dark room visualising calm scenarios is a great way to relax. But it won't help you on the spot, in a stressful situation where you have to be alert and keep functioning but desperately need to calm down.

When you go back to hospital for a follow up, or read another bad news article about cancer, or face another scan or blood test you need a quick technique that can be done anywhere, any time. When you feel tense your breathing rate increases (see fight–flight response, page 36). So, the quickest and most effective way to calm yourself down is to slow your breathing.

How to do slowed breathing

This is not rocket science: the basic idea is just to breathe out for longer than you breathe in:

1. Slowly breathe in **through your nose** to a count of 4. Hold your breath for 3. Then breathe out **through your mouth** for a count of 7 or so.

2. You've probably already forgotten the numbers but they don't matter too much. Just remember: breathe in through the nose, hold your breath for a moment or two then breathe out through the mouth – for about twice as long.

3. As you breathe out, try to let your body go loose and floppy.

4. Repeat this breathing pattern a few times then let your breathing settle into its natural pattern again. It really is as simple as that.

When to use slowed breathing

This skill is great in a highly stressful situation, for example when you're going in to see your medical team for a follow up. This is a situation where you need to express yourself, to hear what is being said and to retain information. You can't afford to be overwhelmed by anxiety. Nor can you afford to be distracted by complicated relaxation routines. Slowed breathing is ideal because it's simple and quick. It allows you to gain control over your body and mind so you can focus on what's really important.

Slowed breathing: Some useful add-ons

If you are in a situation where it's possible to pay a bit more attention to the relaxation skill (for instance sitting in the waiting area before meeting your medical team), there are a few add-ons to slowed breathing that can help deepen the relaxation.

- **Observe your body**: Notice how your shoulders rise with your in breath. Pay attention to your shoulders as they drop back down with the out breath.

- **Loosen up**: Encourage this natural loosening of muscles around your shoulders. Imagine the relaxed feeling from your out breath spreading down your arms, down the trunk of your body and out through your legs.

- **Talk to yourself (in your mind)**: On the out breath say to yourself words such as 'calm', 'quiet', 'loose', 'warm' and 'heavy'. Try to imagine these feelings flowing through your body. Or, try repeating a coping statement or instruction to yourself, such as 'I'm OK', 'I am focused', 'Keep calm', 'Slow down', 'Unwind'.

- **Focus on the 'here and now'**: Keeping the anxious thoughts out of your mind can be incredibly hard in a stressful situation. Focusing on the immediate details of your environment can be a good antidote to racing thoughts. Try really focusing on a particular part of the room: a smudge on the wall, a pattern on the floor. Examine it in enormous detail – colours, shapes, textures. Your mind is likely to wander, but don't judge yourself when it does, just bring your focus back to the area you're concentrating on.

Skill 2: Muscle squeeze–release

This is a deeper form of physical relaxation where you tense your muscles first, then release the tension, leaving your muscles surprisingly relaxed.

Try this right now: clench your fists tightly for five to ten seconds – then release. You'll notice a significant difference between the tensed muscles and the released muscles. When you have released them, you have relaxed them!

How to do it

Overall, try not to get hung up on techniques with this one. Again, there's no magic formula. **But if you feel any pain at any point then stop using that muscle group.** Muscle squeeze–release is about creating and noticing a level of tension, it is not about pain.

You can find your own way to tense then release each muscle, but if you do want a pattern, this one works really well:

1. **Get into a comfortable position**, sitting down or lying is fine. You can do it standing up, but it's probably better to 'graduate' to this, once you've learned the technique.

2. **Fists**: Clench your fists for a few seconds, feel the tension around your hands and lower arms. Release the tension and feel the relaxation flowing in.

3. **Elbows**: Pull your elbows into your sides, hunch your shoulders up towards your ears, feel tightness in the muscles of your upper arms, shoulders and upper back. Hold for a few seconds and then release. Feel the tension go and relaxation flow in.

4. **Chin**: Pull your chin to your chest, clench your teeth and frown. This tightens the muscles of your neck and face. Focus on how hard they're working, pulling against each other, clenching tight and tense. Release and feel the muscles loosening, unwinding and becoming smooth, soft and supple.

5. **Tummy**: To tighten the muscles of your abdomen you can either pull your tummy in or push it out, and hold it there. Whatever you do, feel the muscles pulling tight and tense, working hard to hold the position. Then release, and feel the rush and relief of relaxation.

6. **Buttocks**: Clench your buttocks and hold. Imagine the muscles all scrunched up tight. Release and imagine the muscles smoothing out, loosening and unwinding.

7. **Thighs/upper legs**: Do them one at a time. Lift one leg from the chair/bed/floor and hold for a few seconds. Feel the muscles working hard. The leg may even wobble a bit. Let it down, let the tension go and feel the relief of relaxation replacing the tension. Repeat with the other leg.

8. **Lower legs**: You can do these at the same time. Pull your toes forward, as if towards your face and feel the stretch in the back of your calves. Notice a gentle pulling and stretching in your lower leg and calf muscles. Imagine they are like an elastic band and as you release, feel the tension rushing out to be replaced by relaxation.

Now give yourself a few minutes to enjoy the warm, heavy, loose feeling in your body. With your out breath release any leftover tension.

How to develop the muscle squeeze–release

Over time, perhaps a month or so after you've regularly practised the muscle squeeze–release, you could start to bring the separate areas of your body together, as you squeeze–release the muscles. For example, you could shift to thinking about your body in sections: upper, mid and lower. Tense and release your upper body (using 2, 3 and 4, in the list above, at the same time). Then do your mid body (5 and 6 together). Finally, do your lower body (link 7 and 8).

As you feel more and more confident you can adapt muscle squeeze–release to suit your needs, either taking loads of time over it and really luxuriating in how relaxed your body gets, or developing a 'whole body' muscle squeeze–release that you can do for instant relaxation any time any place. Or you could do both, whenever suits you.

> **TIP ▶**
>
> ### BE SELECTIVE IF YOU WANT
>
> If there's a part of your body that you feel anxious about or uncomfortable about focusing on, then it's fine to leave that body part out of this exercise. Once you feel more confident you might want to bring it in. But don't worry if you can't.

When to use the muscle squeeze–release

Basically use it whenever you want or need to – whatever works for you. Remember there are no 'right' ways to do this; there are no side effects if you don't follow the instructions, no moments when it's wrong to try it. So just test it out and see what it can do for you in different situations. Here are some suggestions to start with:

1. **Last thing at night** as a way of releasing the physical tensions that have built up. Bring it into your wind down time (see Chapter 7: Sleep, page 215).

2. **First thing in the morning** as a way to face the day feeling physically relaxed and mentally calm. This can be particularly helpful if you've had a disturbed night.

3. **After a stressful situation**: Taking a few minutes (even just two or three although ten might be better) to do the muscle squeeze–release after a hospital visit, job interview, difficult conversation, seeing your bank statement, can help you to release some muscle tension, calm racing thoughts and decide what to do next.

4. **During a stressful situation**: This may take some working out (you're unlikely to be able to do the whole, slow body exercise!) but elements of muscle squeeze–release can come in handy during difficult situations. For instance if you're stuck in a traffic jam you can grip the steering wheel, hunch up your shoulders, grit your teeth – then release. Sitting waiting for a medical check-up you could clench your buttocks, pull in your tummy, tense your thighs, then release.

5. **As a way to help you to get off to sleep.** This is slightly different from making it part of your wind down time. During wind down time you can do it in a bath, an armchair, on the sofa. The idea is to release the physical tightness and tension that builds up during the day and give yourself 'quiet time'. But if you are using muscle squeeze–release to fall asleep, you need to do it in bed, last thing. You can also deepen it, by adding in other

relaxation techniques, such as slowed breathing or visualisation (see page 243).

CASE STUDY

Harold, 72, prostate cancer survivor

Harold aimed to put his cancer experience firmly behind him. He didn't like talking about it and found that on the whole keeping himself busy during the day worked well. But he found it very difficult to sleep at night.

It wasn't racing thoughts or worries that disturbed him; he just felt very tense – what he described as 'over tired' – by the time he went to bed. He had mobility problems, and so my suggestions about getting out of bed if he was lying awake for too long were not possible for him. However, muscle squeeze–release worked brilliantly for him. Harold enjoyed the feeling of having more control over his body. He used this relaxation skill every night, and over time he adapted the exercises so that he could tense his whole body in one go, then release it. He loved the feeling of letting his whole body relax all at once. He found that, on the whole, it was much easier to get off to sleep at night after he'd done this. And on the nights when he still couldn't sleep, he was less distressed and more relaxed. As a consequence, he felt better the following morning.

'I like how simple it is,' he told me. 'I don't have to think, and it's such a release that, even if I don't fall asleep then and there, I feel instantly calmer. I have now become such a fan of it that I use it in the day as well. I had a problem getting my pension money out of the post office last week and instead of getting worked up I did my whole body squeeze, went back to the counter and sorted it out.'

TIP▶

ENHANCED MUSCLE SQUEEZE–RELEASE FOR SLEEP PROBLEMS

After you've done muscle squeeze–release, if you still aren't asleep, try to focus on the feeling of heaviness and relaxation. Enjoy the feeling of sinking into your pillow and mattress. You can also add in a visualisation exercise (see below). Try to make your visualisation focus on sleep: maybe you're lying under a sun umbrella on a tropical beach, or curling up under a luxurious feather duvet in a four-poster bed. It helps to plan your sleep images in advance. Think of yourself as a kind of film director – you wouldn't kick off filming without a clear plan and a script developed in advance – well, this works the same way. Direct your own calming movie.

Skill 3: Visualisation

This is a mind relaxation technique that doesn't use the body. It's a classic skill – the sort of thing most people think of when you say 'relaxation method' – because it actually does involve taking yourself off to your fantasy desert island (or some other nice place) in your mind.

When to use visualisation

You can combine visualisation with other, more physical, skills – it will deepen your calm when you've already done slowed breathing or the muscle squeeze–release. You might be able to do it if you have to wait around and are feeling tense, or you could do it later, when you get home from a stressful event. If, after some practise (say five minutes most days for a week or two), you find that you like visualisation, it can almost become a little reward – you go off into your head for a little bit, perhaps when you're having a sit down and a cup of tea after a bout of activity.

Making visualisation work for you

It's important to think carefully about your visualisation before you start. Be the film director. You want to find the imaginary 'place' that really works best to calm you down.

To do this, ask yourself:

1. **What makes me tense?** Is it an 'overload of tasks' or other people's demands, or your own expectations, or fear of the cancer coming back, or loud noises, big crowds, being alone? For example, if you get tense when overloaded by tasks or demands imagining yourself lying flat on a beach might be too extreme a leap. If you're a very active person the idea of just lying still might actually wind you up even more. If so, you could imagine walking along a tropical beach hunting for shells, or swimming through the waves, feeling your body supported by the water. Similarly if you hate being alone, then the notion of lying on a deserted tropical beach might fill you with tension. Maybe a crowded beach in Spain, with chatter and laughter, people throwing balls and splashing would work better? Basically, just find something that works for you – an imaginary place that you do find relaxing.

2. **What does my body do when I'm tense?** Do you feel hot, fidgety, buzzing – or do you slow down? If you get hot when tense, then it might not be a good idea to imagine yourself on a sun-drenched desert island. You might be better off in a cool, shady wood, or on a breezy beach. You could even picture yourself in a comfortable cosy place in your own home. In short,

then, this 'idealised' image of a luxurious desert island might not work that well for you. The key is to keep it personal.

VISUALISATION PLACES

Here are some examples of places that other cancer survivors have found useful in their visualisations:

- an imaginary tropical island beach
- an infinity pool on an Italian hillside
- a Scottish sea loch with lapping waves and majestic mountains behind
- a bluebell wood in May with dappled sunlight illuminating the leaves of the trees and a carpet of bluebells underfoot
- a campsite by a lake
- a snow-capped alpine mountain
- a flower garden in the local park
- the deck of the ferry to a well-loved holiday destination
- a favourite childhood tree house
- the grandparents' home, visited during childhood
- the local swimming pool
- the back garden
- an allotment
- a favourite art gallery
- a luxurious double bed
- a favourite armchair in the living room.

How to do it

The idea is to distance yourself from your immediate surroundings. Clearly, this technique isn't much good for times
when you need to be alert – in traffic jams, or talking to your
medical team. But it's a great way of giving yourself a bit of
'time out' once that tricky moment has passed. Again, there is
no set method here. It does help to begin with a bit of slowed
breathing or muscle squeeze–release, but some people just
leap straight into visualisation without preparation and it
works fine.

1. **Find your place in your mind and see it as clearly as
   you can**: Where are you? What can you see?

2. **Now use all your other senses**: What are the sounds,
   smells, tastes, feel of your place? If you use all your
   senses the visualisation becomes engrossing, detailed and
   soothing, and it will last longer.

EXAMPLE

Flower garden

Say you're in the flower garden of your local park: imagine
the layout of the flowerbeds, the colour of the flowers, the
hedges surrounding them, the people walking through.
Then think about what you can hear – a snatch of bird
song, the scrunch of gravel, toddlers chattering, and distant
traffic. What can you feel? Your clothes on your body, the
temperature of the air around you – imagine yourself
walking through the flower garden with the gravel or
tarmac underfoot, the warm (or cool) breeze as it touches
your skin. . . What can you smell? The scent of the flowers
drifts over you – can you differentiate the rose from the lily?
Is the grass newly mown? Do you get a whiff of perfume as

someone walks by you? Finally, bring in your sense of taste: Are you sucking a mint? Licking an ice-cream? Sipping a coffee? Does the smell of the flowers almost give you a taste sensation in your mouth?

TIP▶

GIVE IT TIME

Don't expect this to come together immediately. This level of visualisation takes time and practice to develop. It's worth the effort, but it's not always achievable. Even those who are really good at visualisation will have days when they just can't get it. You might be distracted by things going on around you in real life, or you might find that the images you've conjured up keep changing. If this happens, don't worry. It's normal. Try changing your image (you don't have to have only one visualisation place to try: the more the merrier). You can also try to simply bring your mind back to your image again – don't judge yourself for feeling distracted. It's OK. Just focus again. If none of this works, just leave it for that moment. Next time it might work better.

CASE STUDY

Linda, 60, breast cancer survivor

Cooling visualisation

Linda had successfully completed her active treatment four years before she came to see me. She was coping very well, working full time as a business woman, married. However in the run-up to her six-monthly check-up she'd get really anxious.

→

She'd get hot flushes and would blush during each follow-up appointment. The flushes and blushing also happened at other stressful times, such as board meetings or during public speaking events.

She couldn't stop focusing on her own heat and skin colour. When meeting her consultant, she couldn't concentrate properly on the discussions. Her consultant commented that she seemed distracted and anxious, and after they'd talked a bit, he suggested that she meet me.

Linda wanted to learn relaxation techniques to help her cope with stressful situations. She found that talking herself through the slowed breathing technique before a work or hospital appointment was very helpful. But what she really took to was visualisation.

When Linda felt her skin temperature rise, she immediately did her slowed breathing and followed this with an image of herself splashing in a mountain stream. She became so skilled at this that when she didn't have time to take even a minute out to visualise (for instance, when talking to her consultant), she'd imagine that her hand was trailing in the cool mountain stream. Then, when she rubbed her face, she'd feel the cool water on it. This 'quick fix' version of visualisation took a lot of practice, but it considerably reduced the problem. Linda's anxiety about the flushes and heat almost totally disappeared and she was far more able to concentrate on the matter in hand.

Skill 4: Mindfulness

This technique has its origins in Buddhism (though don't let that alarm you). It combines relaxation with simple meditation skills that enable you to focus on the 'here and now', rather than fretting and thinking ahead (or back). This is not airy-fairy stuff: there is solid scientific evidence to show that mindfulness is a useful psychological tool for coping with difficulties after cancer.

The idea is pretty simple: going over past events, or thinking ahead to possible future outcomes contributes significantly to tension, worries or distress. Simply learning how to 'be in the moment' can really help. People who use mindfulness say that it gives them a much greater sense of peace and calm, whatever stresses they are facing.

With mindfulness you learn to:

- move away from making judgements about your own thoughts and behaviour (as well as other people's)
- just observe yourself, your thoughts and your reactions, as and when they are happening
- tune into the 'here and now', by focusing on your senses – vision, sound, taste and touch.

Mindfulness, in other words, is not about trying to get anywhere or to feel anything special. It's about observing what's happening, without judging it.

TIP▶

JUST NOTICE

You are not going to push thoughts away but you aren't going to examine them this time either. Instead, you're simply trying to notice the thoughts as they happen, and let them be, without judging or inspecting them.

Mindfulness 1: Mindful breathing

Mindful breathing, our first example of the mindfulness technique, is similar to slowed breathing (on pages 236–7), but the emphasis is different. You don't focus on tackling tension. Instead, you focus on the breathing itself – the present moment – while clearing your mind of other thoughts. Sometimes, when you pay attention to your breathing, the breathing itself can change but in this exercise there's no right or wrong way to breathe. You don't make any judgement whatsoever about how you are breathing, or try to change it, you just observe it.

1. Get comfortable and gently let your eyes close.

2. Bring your attention to your tummy, notice how it rises when you breathe in and falls when you breathe out.

3. Let yourself 'go with' your breathing – as if you are riding the waves of your own breath.

4. When your mind wanders off (and it will), simply, and without judging yourself, bring it back to your breathing again. Repeat this as often as you need to – and at first you'll need to a lot!

5. Try to practise this for five to ten minutes every day.

6. Notice how it feels to focus on your breath without having to do anything else.

Mindfulness 2: Food exercise

The idea of this exercise is to show you that when you focus your mind on the detail of the here and now – pay attention to the smallest and simplest things – you generally feel calmer. Some people says this exercise puts them back in touch with childhood – they remember how interested they were in the world around them (think about how long it can take to walk down a street with a toddler who stops to investigate every flower, leaf, brick or bug). Again, this can be very calming.

You'll need a small piece of food, such as a raisin, berry or nut.

1. Hold it, and observe it as if you have never seen it before.

2. Notice how it feels in your hand: Is there any warmth? What are the colour, texture and smell like?

3. Notice any thoughts you have about it, or about this exercise: try to accept these thoughts without making a judgement about them.

4. Bring it towards your lips, keeping yourself aware of how you move. Let it rest on your lips. How does it feel there? Notice how your lips and mouth respond. How does your mouth feel? Where is your tongue? Are you salivating?

5. Put it into your mouth and let it simply rest there for a moment. Notice any urge to chew and then do so, slowly. Be aware of the taste and sensation of it in your mouth. Note the way your mouth responds, the changing texture, the changes in taste as the food moves across your tongue.

6. Watch the impulse to swallow as it approaches. Be aware of how it feels to swallow the chewed-up nut, berry or raisin.

7. Imagine or sense that your body is now one raisin, berry or nut fuller!

When to use mindfulness

Mindfulness 1 and 2 are good exercises for whenever you feel that you want a break from trying to think things through: when you just want 'to be'. Obviously, the skills take time to develop and work. Try not to pressurise yourself with unrealistic expectations. If you do about five to ten minutes most days you should start to see calming benefits within a week or two (though everyone is different and some people take more time than others to develop these skills). If mindfulness sounds interesting to you, there are books and courses that will help you to investigate it further (see recommendation below).

Mindfulness: What next?

If you want to explore mindfulness more, read *Full Catastrophe Living: Using the wisdom of your body and mind to face stress, pain and illness* by Jon Kabat-Zinn (Piatkus, 2001). Kabat-Zinn is a doctor who developed mindfulness as a psychological tool. His books describe the principles of mindfulness very clearly. They will also give you many more practical ways to use mindfulness day to day.

Your 'relax' toolkit

There are countless other relaxation techniques out there, many of which work brilliantly. The ones described here are just a handful – but they're a good handful because they are the easiest to learn without a teacher, and they work. However, if you want to learn more, or are struggling on your own (and many people do) it might be worth finding a relaxation class in your area. Your local cancer support centre will probably run relaxation courses and will be able to advise you about other services that might be useful.

Don't let any old inhibitions hold you back. You've survived something major. You're in a new situation now. And you need new tools if you're going to tackle the challenges you've been left with. You could well discover that things you may have dismissed before – such as meditation, yoga and stretching, or even complementary therapies such as reflexology, aromatherapy or Reiki – give you the boost or release that you desperately need.

Relaxation skills should be a big part of your post-cancer toolkit. Once you get the hang of them, they really will help you to cope far better with anything life throws at you. So do give them a go – you might be surprised at how much better you feel when you do.

Family, friends and carers: How you can help with relaxation

Helping with relaxation: Dos and don'ts

Don't say 'Relax!' Telling someone to relax tends to have the opposite effect. Instead:

Do encourage them to take some time to learn and practise relaxation exercises.

Don't tell them to do a relaxation technique ('Can't you do your deep breathing?') when you see that they're stressed out. You can (both) easily feel cross or lose heart if that doesn't work. Instead:

Do, wherever possible, plan ahead: if you know they'll be facing a stressful scenario, such as a check-up, try to talk beforehand about what techniques they're going to use to tackle their anxiety or tension.

Four more ways to help

1. **Create a relaxing environment:** For instance, you might be able to reduce background noise, put on soothing music, dim the lights or prevent distractions. This will encourage the person to develop the deep relaxation skills outlined in this chapter.

2. **Join in with the relaxation practice:** This can be helpful for both of you, but always check first that they want you there and, if so, whether it's helpful for you to do the exercise at the same time, or whether you'd be better reading out the instructions or acting as time-keeper.

3. **Investigate local resources**: Does the local cancer support centre run relaxation groups? Are there local yoga or meditation classes nearby and, if so, are these suitable for a cancer survivor? It can be hard for a cancer survivor to have to go through their medical history with yet another stranger only to discover that the class isn't suitable for them. You can gather this information so they don't have to (though do check first that they're happy for you to do this research for them).

4. **Make time to relax together**: There is real value in simply relaxing together. Work out what you both enjoy and find soothing – it might be a country walk, visiting an art gallery, going to the cinema, playing cards (not too competitively!), gardening, sitting down for a meal together, watching a favourite TV programme. During this time – and, yes, this bit is easier said than done – try to keep stressful or difficult conversations to a minimum. You may well have many issues to discuss and decisions to make, but get these done another time. Keep your relaxing time relaxed.

CONCLUSION

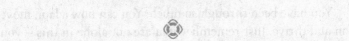

At the very least, this book should have shown you that you are not mad or weak or 'different' because of what you're going through. There are thousands of people wrestling with similar post-cancer emotions right now.

Let's go back to that image from the beginning of this book of your boat in the storm of cancer. It has been damaged, but you now have an emotional recovery toolkit – you can mend it. You also now have the map and provisions that will get you back to shore.

If you've practised any of the exercises already, or even just noticed the odd 'thought trap', then you are on your way. Nobody is expecting you to suddenly feel like your 'old self' again overnight. No one can give you an instant fix or magic you back to the way you were before cancer. But you should now be able to find a new way ahead, that's forward-looking and strong and realistic, and suits you. So, if you haven't thought about where it is you want to get to, then now's the time to start. . .

Nobody can say whether it will take you weeks, months or years to mend your boat and get back to harbour. Your friends and family may have stopped waving; it may feel painfully slow, at times very tricky. But you will get there.

Of course, when you do, the view may be totally different. You may even feel like you're in another country. And as you get stronger, your needs will change: you'll face new challenges, and new emotions. This is why you'll probably need to keep coming back to this book for tips or encouragement, or new exercises to try.

You have been through so much. You can now adapt, move on and thrive. Just remember you are not alone in this – you have at least one companion and it's right here.

RESOURCES

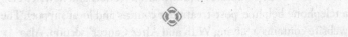

The best place to start when you need more information, support or ideas, is almost always your local health team, either your GP or your hospital cancer team. However, there are plenty of other ways to find support.

Social support

Many cancer survivors find it immensely useful to make contact with people who are going through similar things. National cancer support charities such as Macmillan or Maggie's (see below) or site-specific cancer charities (for instance, organisations such as Breast Cancer Care or the Roy Castle Lung Cancer Foundation) all now recognise how vital post-treatment support is and can connect you with others, both locally and online. Many local organisations can also help you meet other survivors (ask your GP or medical team for details of local organisations).

Support for families and friends

Some cancer support organisations are beginning to recognise that families/friends/colleagues/carers of cancer survivors need support too. Many now have good resources and online chat rooms specifically for those supporting a cancer survivor. You can also ask the medical team at the hospital or your GP for any local groups.

In general, for all aspects of cancer survival these two organisations can be invaluable:

Macmillan Cancer Support

Website: www.macmillan.org.uk

Tel: 0808 808 0000

Offers an online community, information leaflets and newsletters, a telephone helpline, post-treatment courses and local support. The website contains a 'Living With and After Cancer' section. Also provides support for family and friends.

Maggie's Cancer Caring Centres

Website: www.maggiescentres.org.uk

Tel: 0300 123 1801

Offers information and emotional support both from health professionals and other cancer survivors. Also supports family and friends of cancer survivors. Website, information, chat rooms, local drop-in centres close to many UK cancer centres. Runs post-treatment courses.

Online

Cancer Research UK

Website: www.cancerhelp.org.uk

Living Life to the Full

Website:www.livinglifetothefull.com

This is a free online self-help treatment programme, endorsed by the NHS, that helps you to tackle problems such as distress, low mood and worrying, using a practical, step-by-step approach. It is not specifically for cancer survivors, but can help you with many of the issues you are facing.

Further reading on cancer survival

- *The Cancer Survivor's Handbook* by Dr Terry Priestman (Sheldon Press, 2009) covers the areas that our book does not – namely the medical and practical issues facing cancer survivors.

Chapter 1: Worries

To find a therapist try:

British Association of Counselling and Psychotherapy
(BACP) offers information about approved local counselling
services.
Website: www.bacp.co.uk
Tel: 01455 883 300
There are many different kinds of counsellors with different forms
of training, but on the whole their approach is to encourage you to
talk through the difficult situation, explore your feelings and
reactions, make sense of your situation and come to your own
conclusions about how to move forward.

British Psychological Society (BPS) can help you find local
support from trained and accredited psychologists.
Website: www.bps.org.uk
Psychological therapies vary, but in general they tend to be a bit
more structured, with the psychologist taking a more active role in
sessions. If you have been experiencing strong feelings of anxiety,
depression or other distress that have not faded over several weeks
you may find a structured psychological therapy useful.

**British Association for Behavioural and Cognitive
Psychotherapies** (BABCP) will help you find local trained and
accredited cognitive-behavioural therapists.
Website: www.babcp.com
These therapists can be counsellors or psychologists, but they have
undertaken additional training in cognitive behaviour therapy
(CBT). They will help you to understand how your thoughts,
feelings and behaviour are connected, and provide a structured and
practical approach that encourages you to become aware of your
thought processes, challenge unhelpful patterns of thinking, and
find helpful ones instead.

Useful books about worry

- *Overcoming Worry* by Mark Freeston and Kevin Meares (Robinson, 2008)
- *Overcoming Anxiety* by Helen Kennerley (Robinson, 2009)
- *How to Stop Worrying* by Frank Tallis (Sheldon Press, 2009, paperback)
- *Beating Stress, Anxiety & Depression* by Professor Jane Plant and Janet Stephenson (Piatkus, 2008)
- *A Cancer Patient's Guide to Overcoming Depression and Anxiety: Getting through treatment and getting back to your life* by Derek Hopko and Carl LeJuez (US) (New Harbinger Publications, 2008)

Online

Anxiety UK

Website: www.anxietyuk.org.uk

Anxiety UK, Zion Community Resource Centre, 339 Stretford Road, Hulme, Manchester M15 4ZY

Helpline: 08444 775 774

This charity works to relieve and support those living with anxiety by providing information, support and understanding. Also offers one-to-one therapy services and an online members' chat room.

Chapter 2: Depression and low mood

See Chapter 1 resources on how to find a therapist.

For emergency support go to your GP, the accident and emergency department of any hospital or the Samaritans.

Samaritans

Tel: (UK) 08457 90 90 90/(ROI) 1850 60 90 90

Website: www.samaritans.org

A 24-hour, 365-days-a-year telephone helpline. They have particular experience in supporting callers with suicidal or self-harming thoughts.

Useful books about depression

- *Overcoming Depression: A guide to recovery with a complete self-help programme* by Professor Paul Gilbert (Robinson, 2009)

- *Overcoming Depression and Low Mood: A five areas approach* by Dr Chris Williams (Hodder Arnold, revised 2009)

- *Manage Your Mood: How to use behavioural activation techniques to overcome depression* by David Veale and Rob Willson (Robinson, 2007)

- *Mind Over Mood: Change how you feel by changing the way you think* by Christine Padesky and Dennis Greenberger (US) (Guilford Press, 1995)

- *The Mindful Way Through Depression* by Mark Williams, John Teasdale, Zindel Segal and Jon Kabat-Zinn (US) (Guilford Press, 2007)

Online

Mind

Website: www.mind.org.uk

Information line: 0845 766 0163

The mental health charity has excellent online information about depression generally.

Chapter 3: Anger

Again, see Chapter 1 resources for how to find a therapist – many therapists work with anger management.

British Association of Anger Management

Website: www.angermanage.co.uk

4 The Bothy Cottage, Plaw Hatch Hall, Plaw Hatch Lane, Sharpthorne, East Grinstead, West Sussex RH19 4JL

Tel: 0845 130 0286

The British Association of Anger Management offers information about anger, strategies to manage it, group training courses and one-to-one counselling.

Useful books about anger

- *Overcoming Anger and Irritability* by Dr William Davies (Robinson, 2009)
- *Beating Anger: The eight-point plan for coping with rage* by Mike Fisher (Rider, 2005)
- *Taking Charge of Anger: How to resolve conflict, sustain relationships, and express yourself without losing control* by W. Robert Nay (US) (Guilford Press, 2003)
- *Beyond Anger: A guide for men – how to free yourself from the grip of anger and get more out of life* by Thomas J. Harbin (US) (Marlowe & Co., 2000)

Chapter 4: Self-esteem and body image

Useful books about low self-esteem

- *Overcoming Low Self-Esteem* by Dr Melanie Fennell (Robinson, 2009)
- *The Compassionate Mind* by Professor Paul Gilbert (Constable, 2010)

Chapter 5: Relationships and sex

Support for couples

Relate

Website: www.relate.org.uk

Tel: 0300 100 1234

Offers advice, information, relationship counselling and sex therapy both face-to-face, and via online or telephone support.

British Association of Sexual and Relationship Therapy

Website: www.basrt.org.uk

The Administrator, BASRT, PO Box 13686, London SW20 9ZH

Tel: 020 8543 2707

Email: info@basrt.org.uk

A specialist charity for sexual and relationship therapy that offers web-based information and advice and can also help you to find a therapist specialising in sexual and relationship issues.

Institute of Family Therapy

Website: www.instituteoffamilytherapy.org.uk

24–32 Stephenson Way, London NW1 2HX

Tel: 020 7391 9150

The Institute of Family Therapy helps couples or families who are finding relationships problematic and want to explore these issues. The therapy centre is in London but they see many people from outside London. They are experienced in working with families affected by illness and have a sliding scale of charges. Also on offer are mediation and conflict resolution services for families.

Online

Website: therelationshipspecialists.com

You can email one of a specialist team of sex and relationships therapists and get a response in three working days. There is a cost for each enquiry. This can be helpful if you don't feel comfortable with face-to-face consultation.

Support for children and teenagers

Riprap

Website: www.riprap.org.uk

This is a website specifically aimed at children and young people who have a parent with cancer – it offers emotional support, help with understanding your feelings, information about cancer (the website allows you to anonymously ask an expert any question you haven't been able to ask so far). The website also provides contact with others in similar situations and information about what local support is available for you.

Childline

Website: www.childline.org.uk

Helpline: 0800 1111

Provides online and telephone support to children. It also has a website that allows children to get information, chat or email for help and advice.

Useful books about relationship problems

- *Overcoming Relationship Problems* by Michael Crowe (Robinson, 2005)
- *Overcoming Sexual Problems* by Vicki Ford (Robinson, 2010)

Chapter 6: Fatigue

Useful books about fatigue

- *Overcoming Chronic Fatigue* by Mary Burgess with Trudie Chalder (Robinson, 2009)
- *Manage Your Mood* by David Veale and Rob Willson

Online

Website: www.nhs.uk/livewell/

The NHS 'LiveWell' website is a useful guide to all the basics of a good diet and exercise.

Website: www.mayoclinic.com

The Mayo Clinic website is an American site offering a more detailed 'healthy lifestyle' section that covers numerous topics to do with health, exercise and diet.

Chapter 7: Sleep

Useful books about sleep

- *Overcoming Insomnia and Sleep Problems* by Colin A. Espie (Robinson, 2006)
- *Sleepfaring: A journey through the science of sleep* by Jim Horne (Oxford University Press, 2007)
- *Manage Your Mood* by David Veale and Rob Willson – has a useful section on sleep

Online

Website:www.nhs.uk/livewell/
The NHS 'LiveWell' site (see page 264) has some basic insomnia information and tips.

Website:www.sleepfoundation.org
A reliable American website offering a wealth of in-depth information on sleep issues and research. You can also chat online with others who are experiencing sleep problems.

Chapter 8: Relax

Most local cancer support centres (such as Maggie's and Macmillan) run relaxation courses.

Yoga

Yoga is an excellent mind–body exercise that's gentle, relaxing and healing, and can be done by almost anyone. To find a class try your local community centre or go to the British Wheel of Yoga.

British Wheel of Yoga
Website: www.bwy.org.uk
Central Office, British Wheel of Yoga, 25 Jermyn Street, Sleaford, Lincolnshire NG34 7RU
Tel: 01529 306 851

Useful books about relaxation techniques

- *Full Catastrophe Living: How to cope with stress, pain and illness using mindfulness meditation* by Jon Kabat-Zinn (Piatkus, 2001)

- *Wherever You Go, There You Are: Mindfulness meditation for everyday life* by Jon Kabat-Zinn (Piatkus, 2004)

- *Minding the Body, Mending the Mind* by Joan Borysenko (US) (Da Capo, 2007)

- *Mindfulness* by Professor Mark Williams and Dr Danny Penman (Piatkus, 2011)

Relaxation Courses

Online

Website: www.mbct.co.uk

To learn more about Mindfulness-based Cognitive Therapy (MBCT) developed by Mark Williams, Zindel Segal and John Teasdale visit this website. MBCT is based on the Mindfulness-based Stress Reduction (MBSR) eight-week programme developed by Jon Kabat-Zinn.

Stress Management Society

Website: www.stress.org.uk

This is a non-profit organisation, and the website has information about all aspects of stress and ways to cope, from yoga tips to biological information about stress and the brain and silly games to play.

Australia

Australian Cancer Survivorship Centre

Website: www.petermac.org/cancersurvivorship

Peter MacCallum Cancer Centre, Locked Bag 1, A'Beckett Street, East Melbourne VIC 8006

Tel: (03) 9656 1111
Email: contactacsc@petermac.org
Information, help and advice on all aspects of cancer survival,
including information for carers (and health professionals).

Cancer Council

Website: www.cancer.org.au
Helpline: 13 11 20
Information, advice and support for survivors and their carers,
including 'Life after Cancer' forums, 'Cancer Connect' (a free
phone peer support service that puts people in touch with others
who've had a similar cancer experience). Booklets include: 'Life
after Cancer: A guide for cancer survivors'.

CanTeen

Website: www.canteen.org.au
Street Level 6, 235 Clarence Street, Sydney NSW 2001
Free call: 1800 226 833
Email: admin@canteen.org.au
Information and peer support for young people aged 12 to 24
living with (and after) cancer.

Beyond Blue

Website: www.beyondblue.org.au
PO Box 6100, Hawthorn West VIC 3122
Info line: 1300 22 4636
Information and support on all aspects of depression and anxiety –
including information sheets on cancer-related issues – and a
helpline.

Carers Australia

Website: www.carersaustralia.com.au
Tel: 1800 242 636
Offers information and support to carers as well as a carer
advisory and counselling service.

New Zealand

Cancer Society

Website: www.cancernz.org.nz

Operates www.cancerchatnz.org.nz, an online peer support network, and Cancer Connect NZ, a free telephone peer support service. Both resources are for anyone who has been 'touched' by cancer, including carers. Call 0800 226 237 to be put in touch with someone in a similar situation, Monday to Friday, from 9a.m. to 5p.m.

Mental Health Foundation of New Zealand

Website: www.mentalhealth.org.nz

A good way to find resources, information and support for issues such as depression, stress and anxiety.

Carers NZ

Website: www.carers.net.nz

Support and information for carers, including local contacts, factsheets, an email hotline and even carers' radio and TV stations.

USA

Cancer Survivors Network

Website: http://csn.cancer.org/

This is a US-based online network with chat rooms, discussion boards and lots of information for cancer survivors, run by the American Cancer Society. You certainly don't have to be American to find it useful.

INDEX